Clean & Lean
PREGNANCY
GUIDE

THE HEALTHY WAY TO EXERCISE AND EAT
BEFORE, DURING AND AFTER PREGNANCY

James Duigan

James Duigan, world-renowned wellness guru and owner of Bodyism,
London's premier health and fitness facility, is one of the world's
top personal trainers. Bodyism's glittering client list includes
Rosie Huntington-Whiteley, Lara Stone, David Gandy,
Holly Valance, and Hugh Grant.

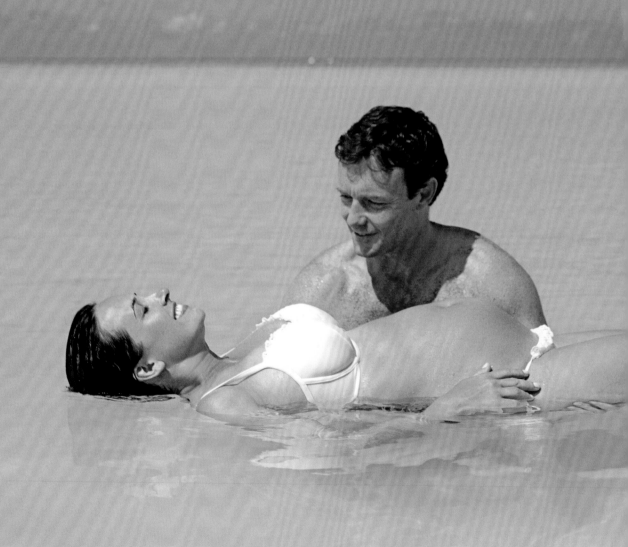

Clean & Lean
PREGNANCY GUIDE

James Duigan

with Maria Lally

Photography by
Sebastian Roos and Charlie Richards

Kyle Books

I'd like to dedicate this book to my beautiful girls, Sophia and Rosie, who I love with all my heart. And to my husband Dan, who is an amazing husband and father. He's the unsung hero of our house and I couldn't do what I do without his love and support.
Maria Lally

Published in 2015 by Kyle Books
www.kylebooks.com
general.enquiries@kylebooks.com

Distributed by National Book Network
4501 Forbes Blvd., Suite 200, Lanham, MD 20706
Phone: (800) 462-6420, Fax: (800) 338-4550
customercare@nbnbooks.com

First published in Great Britain in 2014 by Kyle Books, an imprint of Kyle Cathie Ltd.

10 9 8 7 6 5 4 3 2 1
ISBN 978-1-909487-26-0

Project Editor: Judith Hannam
Copy Editor: Anne Newman
Designer: Dale Walker
Model: Christiane Duigan
Recipe Home Economy: Mima Sinclair
Recipe Styling: Olivia Wardle
Production: Nic Jones, David Hearn and Lisa Pinnell

Library of Congress Control Number: 2014952389
Color reproduction by ALTA, London
Printed and bound in China by C & C Offset Printing Co., Ltd.

The information and advice contained in this book are intended as a general guide. Neither the author nor the publishers can be held responsible for claims arising from the inappropriate use of any remedy or exercise regime. Do not attempt self-diagnosis or self-treatment for serious or long-term conditions before consulting a medical professional or qualified practitioner. Do not begin any exercise program or undertake any self-treatment while taking other prescribed drugs or receiving therapy without first seeking professional guidance. Always seek medical advice if any symptoms persist.

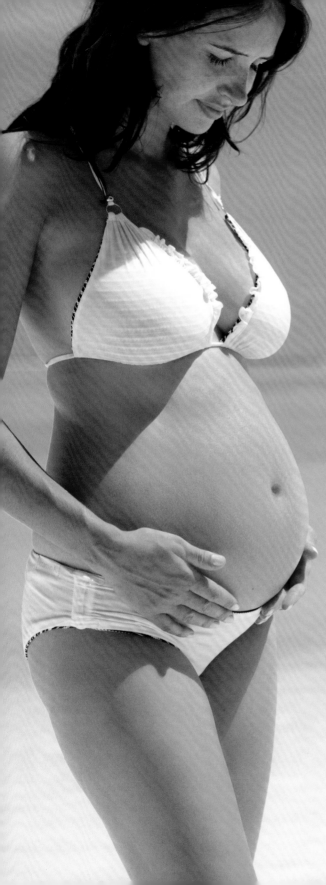

CONTENTS

by Lara Stone

Pregnancy is supposed to be the most amazing time in a woman's life. We've all heard stories of the glowing expectant mom, with the toned legs and neat bump and the instant and deep connection with her unborn baby. I'm sure those pregnancies exist, but mine certainly wasn't like that...

I was in maternity jeans at nine weeks. I was bloated all over, had limp greasy hair, no energy, and I could eat (and waddle) for a village. I felt terrible for feeling this way because I actually had an easy pregnancy—I had no morning sickness, no bleeding, no pain, and my baby and I were perfectly healthy. Yet I didn't get that earth mother feeling I'd been hoping for.

Like a lot of women, I wanted to stay in shape during my pregnancy. But you know what? We're only human. So while we know that we need only an extra 200 calories a day toward the end of the pregnancy, if—like me—you only want to eat deep-fried food, then so be it. The most important thing during pregnancy is to grow a little person inside of you which, when you think about it, is the most amazing miracle in the world.

There is so much pressure these days to look fantastic during pregnancy and to lose the baby weight within days of leaving the hospital. I have nothing against those who do, but it's not normal. Your body changes hugely during a pregnancy and it takes time to go back. My son is now nearly five months old and my body still isn't back to how it was.

I've had lots of ups and downs regarding my body image over the past year. On every level I know I should just be happy to have a lovely healthy baby, and I do count my blessings every day. But seeing articles about me that say, "She's brave to go outside looking like

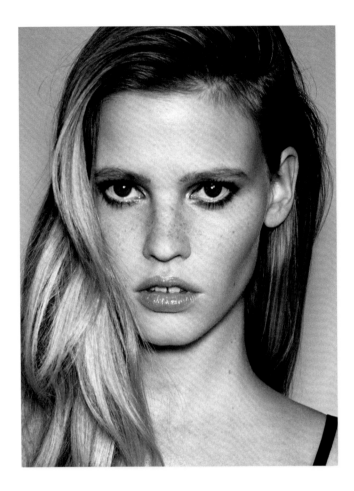

that," "She's struggling with her baby weight," "Is she pregnant again?" or "She can kiss her career goodbye" is painful. And it sends a bad message to other women reading it, who may be feeling bad about their own baby weight.

It's been a struggle to accept the changes in my body but I've eaten Clean & Lean and tried to make time for exercise and I now feel happier, stronger, and more confident. I'm still not in my pre-pregnancy jeans and I'm a few pounds heavier than I was pre-baby, but that's OK. I'm happier than ever and I love every minute of being a mom. And I no longer feel the jealous need to unfollow friends who post bikini selfies ten days after giving birth looking amazing! Because everything is just how it's supposed to be.

INTRODUCTION

I want this book to be your best friend. I want you to feel safe and supported while you read it and I want you to take it everywhere you go so that if you need a little reminder of how amazing you are, or if you need some guidance, it's right there next to you. I want you to share it with your family and I definitely recommend that your partner reads this book as well so you can really experience this journey together.

This book isn't about losing weight, it's about teaching you to be kind to yourself and to focus on your health and the health of your beautiful, precious baby. The good news is when you do this, the weight will fall off effortlessly and you will feel strong, healthy, and vibrant. We've also included guidance and tips to get you through every stage of pregnancy as well as the first 12 weeks after you've given birth.

This is the book Christiane needed when she was pregnant. It has been written to remind you that being pregnant and having a child is a wonderful, natural process, that there is nothing to be afraid of and that what is happening to you is happening to thousands of women all over the world at this very moment. Obviously I'm a man and, as such, I simply can't understand what you're going through as a woman, which is why I've brought together some of the most talented, inspiring, and amazing women in the world to create this book and to provide the blueprint for a happy, safe, and healthy pregnancy and beyond.

We've included stories from beautiful, brave mothers from all over the world and all walks of life. They are there for you to read when you feel lonely and will remind you of the wonderful sisterhood you belong to.

I was Christiane's birth partner and, with the help of our amazing midwife, Julie, I helped deliver our little girl Charlotte. It was the proudest and most "alive" moment of my life. Even now, as I write this, I'm overcome with love and emotion and I have to go for a sobbing, snotty walk to get myself together. Watching my wife go through labor and give birth gave me a deep sense of awe and gratitude. And as I witnessed her holding our newborn child, standing naked, fierce, and beautiful, covered in blood after six hours of primal screams and heroic effort I decided two things; one, this is the strongest most wonderful person I've ever known, one who is truly a warrior. Two, I would never, ever mess with her... ever.

I felt completely at peace as I held my hour-old little girl in my arms and for the first time in my life I knew exactly why I was alive. I felt a deep sense of duty to this little person and I was instinctively and fiercely protective of my family. I loved them both more than I could understand and my father, who had just survived lung cancer, was sitting in the next room waiting to meet the little angel he had stayed alive to see.

Life was good. And then Christiane started to lose blood. A lot of blood. A feeling of helplessness and panic filled every part of me but within seconds, Julie had dealt with the situation and saved Christiane's life. We were lucky and it was in that moment I made a commitment to help as many people come into this world safely and with support. Our beautiful friend Teresa Palmer (Charlotte's Godmother) put us in touch with Christy Turlington and EMC (the Every Mother Counts charity). It is such a blessing to be able to help and contribute to such a wonderful cause that is very close to our hearts.

So please remember that you're not alone, that you are amazing, that you deserve a happy, healthy life, and so does your baby. Thank you for giving me and Christiane the opportunity to help you and share our knowledge and the knowledge and experience of so many wonderful people that have contributed to this book. Sending you lots of love and hugs. And just know this—it's all worth it.

My favorite pregnancy conversation: Me: "Christiane, do you think hormones may be affecting your mood?" Christiane: "No, James, you're just getting more annoying."

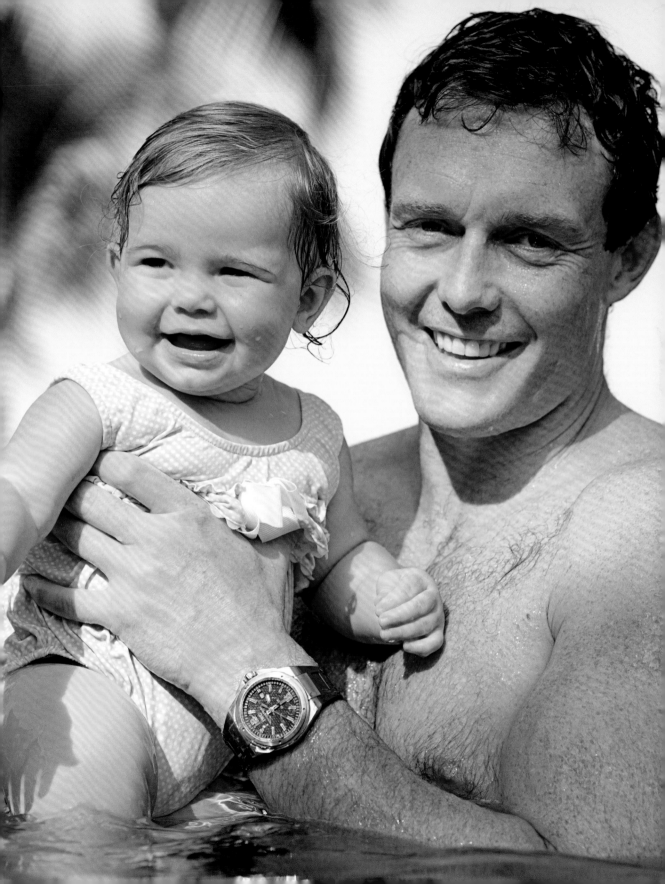

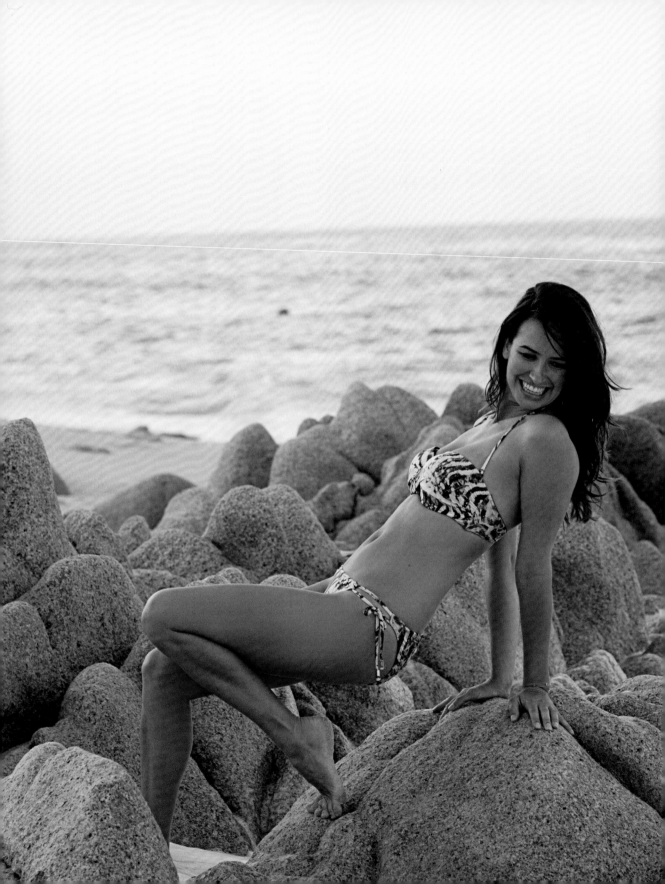

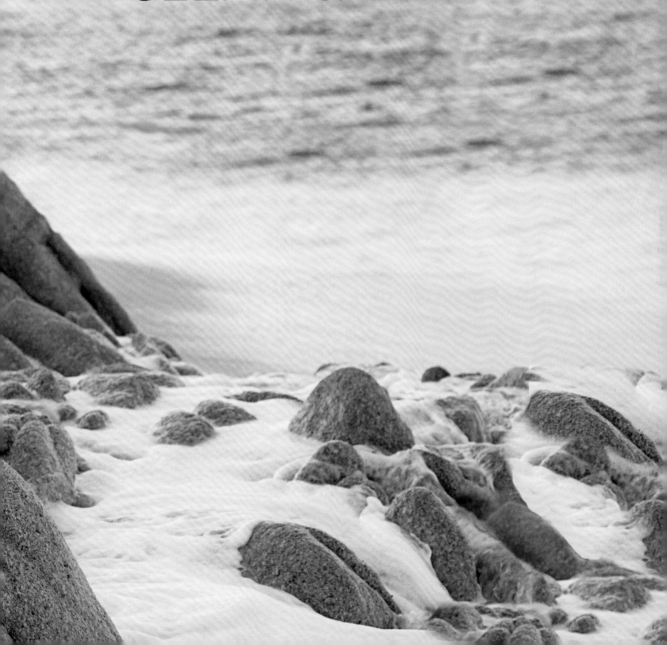

CHAPTER 1

WHAT IS CLEAN & LEAN?

CLEAN & LEAN PREGNANCY

In 2009 I wrote my first book, *The Clean & Lean Diet*. "Clean & Lean" describes the perfect state for your body—"clean" of fattening toxins and "lean" as a result of a nourishing diet and regular exercise. That book became an instant bestseller and I've since written three more about the Clean & Lean way of life: one on how to get a flat tummy, another aimed at men, and a recipe book. And now I bring you Clean & Lean for moms and moms-to-be.

I've spent years working with women who are either trying to get pregnant, trying to stay healthy during their pregnancies, or trying to get back in shape after having one or several babies. Those women—along with supermodel Lara Stone and the actresses Holly Valance and Teresa Palmer, whom I've had the pleasure of training with and knowing for years, and also our great friend Megan Gale—are going to share their stories of pregnancy and motherhood too. Because while it's one thing telling somebody how to stay Clean & Lean, it's another thing telling a new mom—who is sleep, time, and energy deprived, and would rather be bonding with her precious new baby (or sleeping) than exercising.

Good intentions often go out the window when you're tired, craving coffee, and don't have any time for yourself. This really came home to me when my wife Christiane was pregnant with and subsequently gave birth to our beautiful daughter Charlotte in 2012. I saw first-hand just how challenging it can be to eat healthily when you have morning sickness and just want to eat buttered white bread and chocolate all day. Or how difficult it can be to create a nutritious meal when you have a baby on your hip, one hand free, and just five minutes to make breakfast before the next round of feeding and diaper-changing begins.

So I came up with this book—the *Clean & Lean Pregnancy Guide*. It's about self-acceptance, being kind to yourself, and embracing the changes that your body is going through. It's not all about looking great—it's about feeling great. My aim is to take everything I know—from years of experience working with thousands of women all over the world, as well as from watching Christiane get her body back—and help women stay in the best possible shape and feel amazing, but in a realistic way.

So I'm not going to give you complicated healthy recipes that you don't have time to make. Neither am I going to suggest that you try to get back into your jeans six weeks after giving birth because, frankly, it's unlikely and possibly unsafe. Instead, I'm going to give you practical advice that you can follow at your own pace, while enjoying your baby and resting.

This is absolutely not a diet book and I can't stress that enough. No pregnant woman or new mom should be dieting or thinking about restricting their food intake. In fact, when I use the word "diet" in all my books, it doesn't mean what most people think: "diet" is the way you eat, not something you do for a week to lose weight. I want you to change your diet, not "go on" one. We should all change our eating habits so we feel great, pregnant or not. But pregnant women and new moms in particular need to focus on eating wholesome, delicious, nutritious foods that are full of goodness so that they—and their babies—stay healthy and feel amazing. Because if you eat great, you'll feel great, and that's vital when you're facing the physical and emotional challenges of pregnancy and motherhood.

So please don't think of Clean & Lean as a diet in the weight-loss sense. It's a way of eating and a way of living. Let go of guilt and don't concern yourself with "right or wrong" or "good and bad." Simply focus on what works for you and embrace this experience and just celebrate how amazing you are for creating, carrying, and giving birth to new life.

> *If you eat great, you'll feel great, and that's vital when you're facing the physical and emotional challenges of pregnancy and motherhood.*

This book is a blueprint for a happy, healthy pregnancy and a beautiful body. It covers everything from how to increase your chances of getting pregnant, to how to eat and move right in each trimester, to getting your body back afterward and feeling fantastic along the way. **But first, here's a quick reminder of my Clean & Lean philosophy.**

CLEAN & LEAN PHILOSOPHY

In a nutshell, your body will always struggle to be lean unless it's clean. And toxins stored in the body's fat cells will prevent that. If you're dieting, but toxic, your body might lose fat, but these toxins will have nowhere to go except back into your system. You'll feel tired, lethargic, and you may have headaches, which is why most of us feel terrible soon after starting a diet. So if you're toxic, you'll always struggle to lose weight. And ironically, many diets make us more toxic with all their low-fat/high-sugar advice, so the cycle of yo-yo dieting continues.

However, if you stick to "clean" foods, you'll look and feel great. And this is what I mean when I talk about "clean" foods:

✳ They haven't changed much from their natural state. For example, that apple in your fruit bowl looks like it did when it was hanging on the tree. Yet potato chips and bread don't look like they did in the beginning. That's because they've been processed to the point of being unrecognizable. So clean foods are those that haven't been tampered with too much.

✳ They don't have any added fake flavorings, nor are they sweetened with sugary ingredients. Their natural flavor is all that's needed to make them taste great. Succulent steak, in-season greens like asparagus, sweet berries, creamy eggs... clean foods don't need artificial flavors to make them taste good; they're delicious just as they are.

✳ They won't last for months and months. Clean foods develop mold quite quickly because they're natural and not processed with life-lengthening preservatives. A store-bought muffin with a month-long expiration date clearly contains something that's keeping it fresh—that's most definitely not clean.

✳ They don't have a long list of ingredients, many of which you can't even pronounce, let alone recognize. Get into the habit of checking ingredients, reading labels, and avoiding foods that have lengthy ingredient lists. This doesn't take long and isn't difficult—just scan the list and eat only things you know are good for you.

✳ They don't list sugar among their first three ingredients. I'm going to talk a lot about sugar in this book. We're slowly becoming more aware of just how toxic sugar is—it's fattening and makes you tired—and how it's hidden in all sorts of foods. Keep an eye out for it.

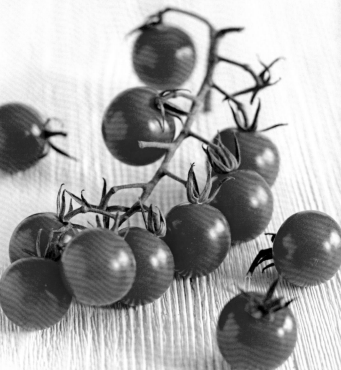

The BASICS

In order to become Clean & Lean, you'll need to familiarize yourself with just a few basic rules.

CUT BACK ON THE CRAP*

*(that's Caffeine, Refined sugar, Alcohol, and Processed foods)

There are four main toxins that cause our bodies to hold on to fat.

C IS FOR CAFFEINE

This is OK in small doses. Even in pregnancy, official guidelines say you can have 200mg of caffeine or one or two cups of coffee a day. High levels of caffeine, however, can result in your baby having a low birthweight, which is associated with an increased risk of health problems later in life. Too much caffeine has also been linked to an increased miscarriage risk. So try not to exceed the 200mg limit per day, and drink plenty of still filtered water instead, because you need to stay hydrated when you're pregnant for your own health and your baby's.

Green tea is full of health-boosting antioxidants. However, it also contains caffeine, so limit yourself to three cups a day and don't drink it at all after lunch as it will disrupt your sleep, which is the last thing you need when you're pregnant or a mom. Another reason I tell clients to limit their caffeine intake is that it can put stress on the body, and when we're stressed, we release a hormone called cortisol which encourages our body to cling to fat.

New moms should also be wary of too much coffee because it can actually make them more tired (I'll talk more about this in Chapter 6). Coffee is also a diuretic—meaning it makes you urinate a lot—which can leave you feeling dehydrated and deplete your body of key

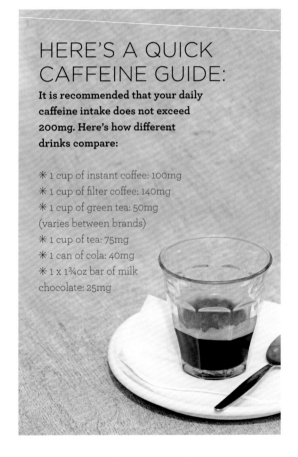

HERE'S A QUICK CAFFEINE GUIDE:

It is recommended that your daily caffeine intake does not exceed 200mg. Here's how different drinks compare:

✳ 1 cup of instant coffee: 100mg
✳ 1 cup of filter coffee: 140mg
✳ 1 cup of green tea: 50mg (varies between brands)
✳ 1 cup of tea: 75mg
✳ 1 can of cola: 40mg
✳ 1 x 1¾oz bar of milk chocolate: 25mg

pregnancy nutrients, like calcium and iron.

It's also a good idea to reduce caffeine intake gradually when you're trying to get pregnant. Switch to decaffeinated teas and coffees and boost your energy levels in others ways: snack between meals (see p. 126 for ideas), do gentle exercise (see Chapter 2), and improve your sleep (see also Chapter 2).

R IS FOR REFINED SUGAR

In a nutshell, sugar makes you fat and tired and even though it often comes in an attractive package (cakes, cookies, chocolate, and carbonated drinks), there really is nothing to love about it. It ages us inside and out and makes us put on weight. In fact, sugar converts to bodily fat faster than fat itself because it raises insulin levels, which in turn causes excess fat to be stored. Studies show that 40 percent of the sugar you eat is converted straight to fat, and that's if you're slim; if you're overweight, up to 60 percent is converted to fat and stored around your stomach, waist, and hips.

As I've already mentioned, sugar makes you tired and, in pregnancy, you feel tired enough already. It leaches vitamins and minerals from your body, too, making you feel hungry and weakening your immune system. A little bit of fresh, homemade cake is fine if you really crave it, but try to avoid consuming a lot of processed sugar in drinks, low-fat yogurts, and sauces on a daily basis.

A IS FOR ALCOHOL

Advice on drinking alcohol in pregnancy changes all the time, but the general consensus is that it's best to avoid it or limit it to very small amounts, such as one to two units a week. I'm not a fan of alcohol in general, let alone in pregnancy, so my take on this one is to avoid it altogether. Why take the risk?

We know that alcohol passes through the placenta and reaches your baby. When you're pregnant, your body also has to work hard to process alcohol out of your system. Excessive alcohol in pregnancy can cause miscarriage, premature birth, and fetal alcohol syndrome (the effects of which can range from learning difficulties to behavioral problems to facial defects and offspring being permanently small for their age). On a lesser note, why drink something in pregnancy that's going to make you feel even more tired and crave more sugar than you already do? Your body is working hard enough during this time, creating a little person, so don't put it under even more stress.

As for new moms who are tempted to have a glass of wine every night to "relax"—I say don't. Alcohol disrupts sleep and causes blood-sugar levels to swing, resulting in tiredness, so it's a bad way to relax. And like caffeine, alcohol puts stress on your system.

Alcohol is also full of sugar and makes you fat around the middle. I call alcohol—especially sugary wine—a "fat bomb" that explodes all over your hips, thighs, stomach, and face. I can always tell when a woman drinks too much because, no matter how slim the rest of her body is, she has "alcohol bloat" around her face and stomach. Remember, too, that the liver is a fat-burning organ, so when it's processing alcohol, it stops burning fat. In short, alcohol leaves you pudgy, so ditch it—or at least (when you're no longer pregnant) cut right back. Find other ways to relax, like resting (when you can), warm baths, gentle exercise, reading, meditation, or music.

P IS FOR PROCESSED FOODS

These go against every Clean & Lean rule there is. The less a food has been altered, the "cleaner" it is. Clean foods include fruit, vegetables, eggs, meat (lean proteins), fish, nuts, and seeds; processed foods, on the other hand, are usually made in factories, stripped of their natural goodness and pumped full of man-made preservatives and additives to make them look appetizing and last longer. So stay away from canned foods, white bread, pasta, and rice, take-out food, most breakfast cereals, and frozen french fries and onion rings. When you're a new mom it's tempting to grab quick foods, but they'll make you more tired because they don't contain enough nutrients. Instead, go for quick and healthy meals—see Chapter 8 for delicious recipes.

MEGAN GALE

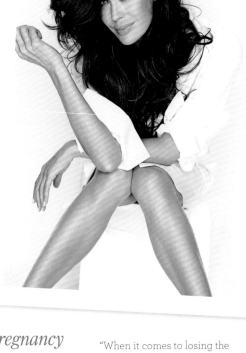

"Before I got pregnant, I had a fairly healthy body image. I've never been super-skinny or overweight—I've just tried to maintain a balance when it comes to food, diet, and exercise. When Shaun and I started trying to conceive I gave up alcohol, although I've never been a big drinker. I also gave up coffee, my biggest vice, even though my midwife has said one to two cups of coffee a day is acceptable. However, with coffee I think it's always good to limit it if you can.

"I'm really enjoying the whole experience of being pregnant, even when I don't feel so great! I had a bit of nausea at the six-to-eight-week mark and felt exhausted. Then I got a cold, then flu, went on antibiotics, and then had a chest infection which hung around until week 13. I'm now 15 weeks and feel much better, but if I've had a busy day my belly starts to feel swollen and heavy, which I think is baby's way of telling me to take it easy, so when it happens I take some time out and just rest.

"People ask whether I find it hard, as a model, to watch my body change. But I just find it mind-blowing to discover what our bodies are capable of. Like most women, I find some days it can be hard to get your head around the weight gain and expanding waistline. But I just remind myself why it's happening and how wonderful that reason is. It's also a reminder of how primal we really are. During pregnancy and motherhood, a woman's intuition is at an all-time high, so try to tap into that and instinctively do what feels right for you.

During pregnancy and motherhood, a woman's intuition is at an all-time high, so try to tap into that and instinctively do what feels right for you.

"When it comes to losing the baby weight, women are often in a lose/lose situation. Especially women in the public eye—if they carry the baby weight for too long, they're criticized for losing their figure. If they get back to their pre-baby shape too quickly, it's implied they've been excessively dieting and exercising and are obsessed with being thin again and not thinking about their baby. They can't win. And I'm not even going to concern myself with any of that—I'm just going to concentrate on bonding with my baby.

And I can't wait!"

FAT DOESN'T MAKE YOU FAT

Don't be fat phobic! There are different types of fat: good, clean fats are the heart-friendly kind found in nuts, avocados, oily fish, and oils; bad fats are found on the edge of a slice of bacon, speckled through a processed meat, or in a pie crust, for example, and they should be avoided. So when I say eat more fat, I mean good fat. Good, clean fats should be eaten every day. For one thing, they help your body to absorb vitamins and minerals more efficiently, and this is incredibly important during pregnancy. For this reason, always add good fat to a salad, as it'll help your body to absorb all the goodness from the lettuce, peppers, and cucumbers. Good fats also reduce sugar cravings, lift your energy levels, improve your ability to concentrate, and keep you feeling full for longer. And as if all that weren't enough, they also plump up your skin and make your hair shine. In pregnancy, omega-3 fatty acids—found in oily fish—also help your baby's brain development.

WHERE ARE TOXINS FOUND?

* Sugar
* Alcohol
* Carbonated drinks
* Processed food
* Processed "diet" food
* Excess caffeine

*top tip

While you are pregnant, try to only have organic whole milk because other milks can contain growth hormones and antibiotics, which can be passed on to your baby!

WHAT ABOUT VEGETARIANS?

Clean & Lean is easy for vegetarians. Simply include lots of vegetarian proteins in your diet such as legumes, beans, lentils, and chickpeas, and rather than rely too heavily on bread and pasta, choose grains such as quinoa, oats, and wild rice. Also have lots of good fats from avocados, walnuts, pecans, almonds, Brazil nuts, and sesame, flax, and pumpkin seeds.

So that, in a nutshell, is what Clean & Lean is. It's a fairly simple way of eating and living. Just remember—if it didn't once fly, swim, or walk, or wasn't pulled from the ground, from a bush, or a plant, don't eat it! And you don't have to get this right 100 percent of the time; if you aim for just 80 percent, you'll be OK.

As I'll explain over the next eight chapters, during pregnancy, more than ever, you need to listen to your body. But remember, if you're pregnant, everything you eat, drink, and do, your baby is experiencing too. I'm not saying that to make you feel guilty—I'm saying it so you'll treat your own body and health during pregnancy in the same way as you'll treat your baby's once they are born. You want only the best for them, so they feel good and grow up healthy, and you need to treat yourself just as kindly. It's the same for new moms—I've seen so many who feed their baby puréed organic vegetables, while they have coffee and chocolate themselves.

You deserve to be looked after too and that's what this book is all about. Good luck!

CLEAN & LEAN FOODS

CLEAN & LEAN PROTEINS

Great sources of protein:
* Chicken
* Turkey
* Lamb
* Beef
* Duck
* All fish (but remember: just two servings of oily fish a week in pregnancy and no shark, marlin, or swordfish; try to limit tuna as well)

And for vegetarians:
* Eggs
* Beans
* Lentils
* Nuts
* Seeds
* Yogurt
* Cheese

*top tip

Freeze your fruit! Wash and cover bite-sized pieces of fruit—such as whole grapes and blueberries, halved strawberries, and chunks of pineapple—and place in the freezer. When you feel like something sweet or crave ice-cream or a popsicle, try some frozen fruit instead to satisfy your sweet craving.

CLEAN & LEAN FLAVORS

The more fresh flavors you put into your food, the better it will taste and the easier it will be to avoid all those nasty fake flavors in the form of processed sugar and additives. **Here are some ideas:**

* Avocado oil
* Basil-infused oil
* Coconut oil
* First-press extra virgin olive oil (the best that you can buy)
* Flaxseed oil
* Sesame oil
* Walnut oil
* Garlic-infused olive oil
* White wine vinegar
* Delouis Fils mayonnaise (keep refrigerated)
* Dijon mustard
* Tamari (gluten- and sugar- and salt-free)
* Lemons
* Limes
* Garlic
* Cilantro
* Dill
* Oregano
* Parsley
* Thyme
* Chile
* Cinnamon
* Cayenne pepper
* Turmeric

And here are some of my own personal favorite flavors that deserve a special mention:

* Cinnamon can reduce blood-sugar levels and, therefore, sugar cravings and bad cholesterol. It's also an anti-inflammatory, so it can help with aches and pains. Sprinkle ground cinnamon in your coffee or over your oatmeal.
* Garlic helps with so many things. It's antiviral, so it wards off colds and boosts your immune system, plus it's an antioxidant and lowers bad cholesterol.
* Ginger is a great antioxidant. It's also been shown to boost the immune system, help blood circulation, and aid digestion. Slice some of the root into hot water with a squeeze of lemon to make a refreshing drink.
* Parsley helps the kidneys flush out toxins, plus it freshens your breath. It's also good for keeping blood-sugar levels steady.
* Rosemary is great for your brain and is used by aromatherapists the world over to improve mood.

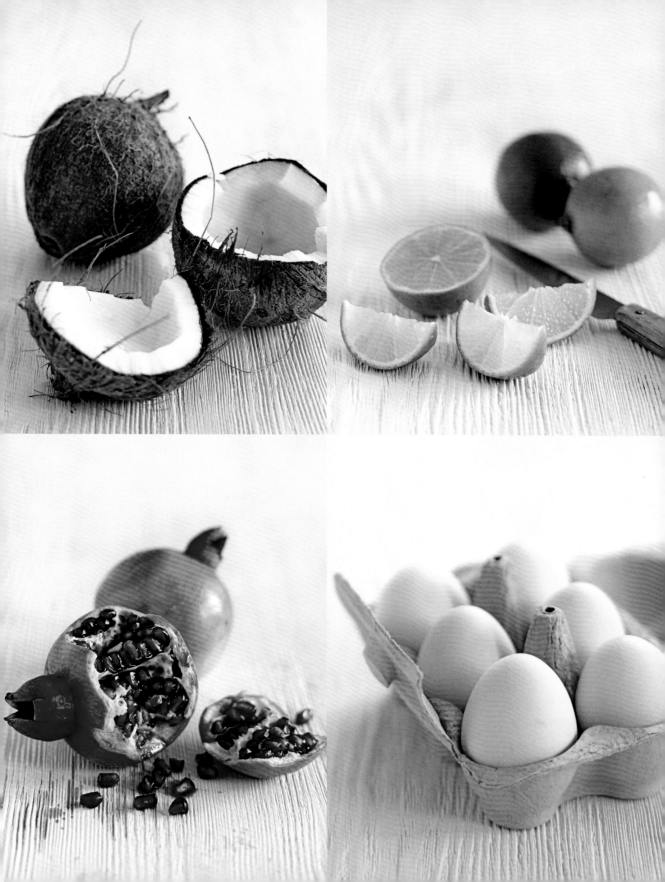

CLEAN & LEAN VEGETABLES

Vegetables that are organic and in season contain twice as many vitamins as those that are not. Try local farmers' markets, and if you can't afford to buy organic, always try to buy in-season. Out-of-season vegetables have often been flown for miles, so are sprayed with life-lengthening preservatives and may contain fewer nutrients.

The following vegetables are good choices:

- Arugula
- Asparagus
- Avocado
- Bell peppers
- Broccoli
- Brussels sprouts
- Butternut squash
- Carrots
- Cauliflower
- Cucumber
- Green beans
- Kale
- Snow peas
- Spinach
- Sweet potato
- Watercress
- Zucchini

CLEAN & LEAN NUTS & SEEDS

Eat raw nuts whenever possible—the roasting process can cause nuts to go rancid, which increases free-radical damage in your body. Try the following:

Nuts
- Almonds
- Brazil nuts
- Cashews
- Chestnuts
- Macadamia nuts
- Peanuts
- Pecans
- Pistachios
- Walnuts

Seeds
- Chia
- Flax
- Linseed
- Pumpkin
- Sesame
- Sunflower

*top tip

Make a big portion of your favorite meal, divide it up into containers, and keep some in the fridge and some in the freezer—perfect for those days (and especially evenings) when you're too tired to cook, but want something filling and nutritious.

TRY THIS DIP

Mash up and mix half an avocado, a dollop of full-fat Greek yogurt, some crushed garlic, chopped fresh cilantro, chopped jalapeño pepper, lime juice, ground cumin, salt, and pepper. Eat on its own or with gluten-free crackers or rye bread.

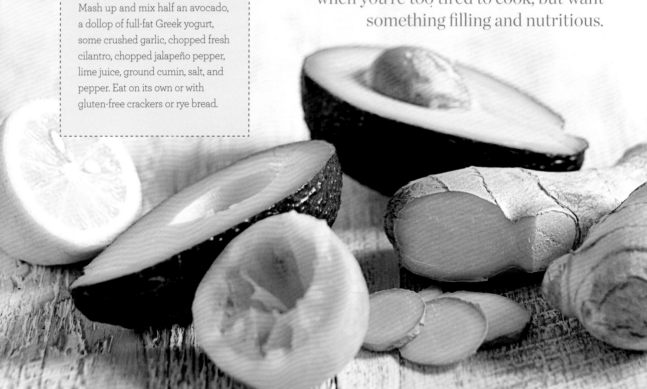

TERESA PALMER

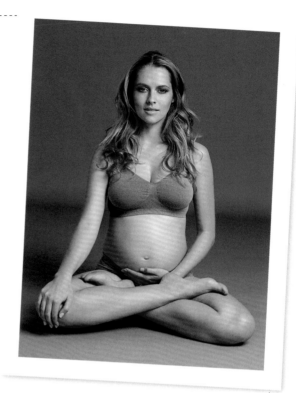

"Ever since I was a little girl all I've longed for is to become a mother. I had an old-fashioned pram and I filled it with dolls and lugged it around everywhere. Now I'm 27 and expecting my first child, a son, with my husband Mark.

"It took us seven months to get pregnant, which doesn't sound like a long time. But it felt like an eternity, as anybody who has tried, or is trying, to get pregnant will know. I'd spent my whole adult life trying not to get pregnant but then, when I wanted to, it wasn't that easy. I was disappointed with my body and felt a lot of despair.

"Once I was pregnant, the self-judgment didn't stop. I placed huge expectations on myself and felt guilty if I ate something 'bad.' Before I got pregnant I told myself I'd be the healthiest pregnant woman ever—nothing processed and nothing fried would pass my lips. But I was shocked to discover that's exactly what I craved—I just wanted fries and sweets!

"Pregnancy wasn't at all how I'd expected it to be. But that's the problem right there—placing an expectation on how things 'should' be. Once I freed myself from expectation, I began to enjoy my pregnancy and the changes it brought. I marveled at the aches and pains I experienced and my protruding belly. Once I sat back and allowed the experience of pregnancy to come to me—without trying to control it—I felt more rooted. It's the art of surrendering—observing your body and trusting it to tell you what it needs.

"I didn't exercise at all during the first trimester—I was too exhausted and chose sleep instead because I listened to my body. After 12 weeks, I started Pilates and yoga. It was beautiful to regain some strength. I freed myself from guilt about what I ate too, and had what I wanted but in a

Once I allowed the experience of pregnancy to come to me, I felt more rooted. It's the art of observing your body and trusting it to tell you what it needs.

mindful way. I had a green juice every day and a plant-based prenatal vitamin supplement, so if I made a few unhealthy diet choices, they balanced things out.

"The day we saw our little man doing somersaults on the ultrasound scan was the most special feeling I've ever had. We had created this little being! And those tiny toes we were watching wriggling on the screen were the very same toes we would be kissing in a few months' time. It bought home to me just how miraculous a journey pregnancy is. It's so special, so surreal, and yet so natural.

"Lastly, I believe all women have the right to have birthing options and be able to have their best birth possible. Whichever path you choose—medicated, non-medicated, in a hospital environment or at home—you know how best to birth your own baby."

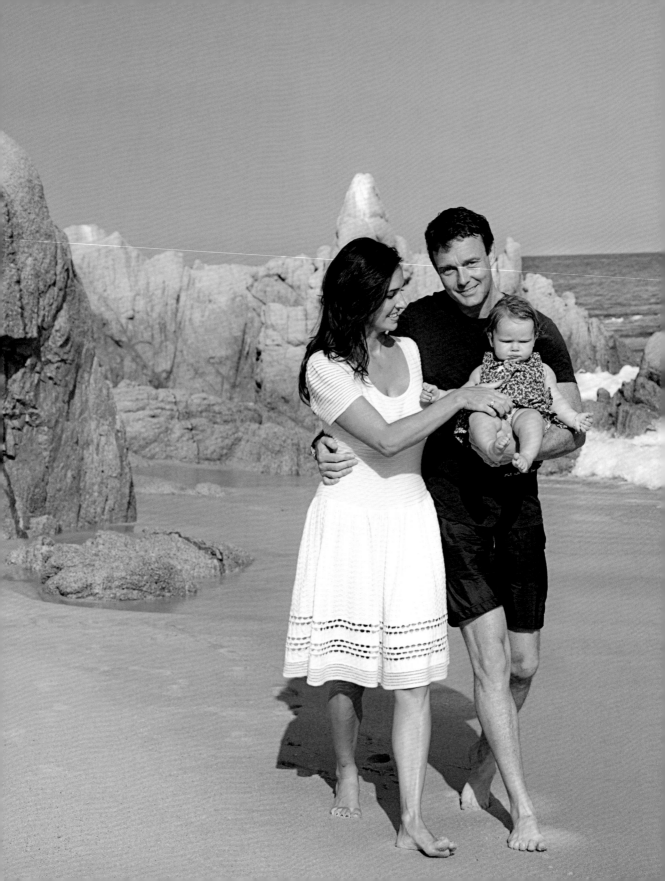

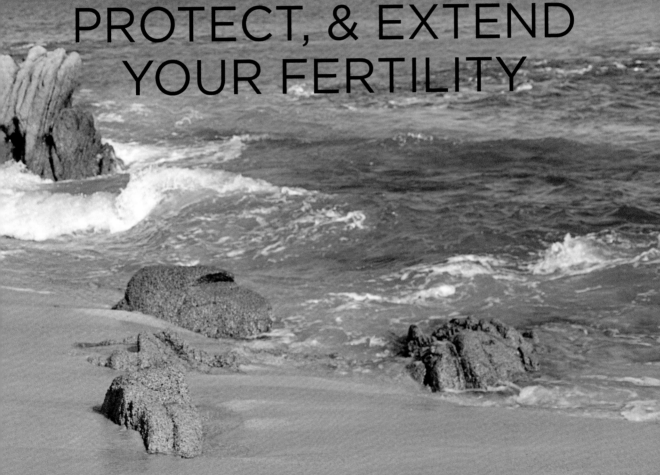

CHAPTER 2

HOW TO BOOST, PROTECT, & EXTEND YOUR FERTILITY

I couldn't write a book about pregnancy without addressing the fact that getting pregnant in the first place isn't easy for everybody. Nothing brought this home to me more than when my wife Christiane and I struggled to conceive our daughter Charlotte. We were both young and healthy, so took our fertility for granted, never imagining it could take so long.

There is still so much to discover about why some people become pregnant easily and others don't. But what we do know is that there are several steps you can take to help you along the way. As Christiane and I prove, being healthy isn't a guarantee of fertility, but countless studies do link a healthy lifestyle to increased fertility, so making the right changes to your life could improve your chances. And taking control of your fertility is important, because when you're trying and failing to conceive, you often feel powerless.

So this chapter, based on a combination of my work with clients who were trying to get pregnant, our own experience, and the advice of some fantastic experts we met during that time, is my guide to increasing, protecting, and extending your fertility.

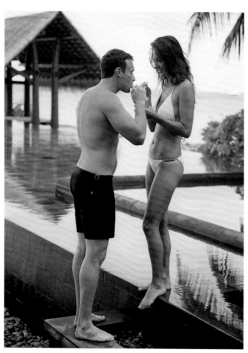

INFERTILITY EXPLAINED

Jane is a world-renowned fertility specialist and Clinical Director of the Acupuncture IVF Support Clinic (www.acupunctureivf.com.au). She helps couples going through IVF to conceive with the help of Chinese herbs and acupuncture and she's amazing—she supported Christiane and me through a very difficult time. There are some experts who just stand out and Jane is one of them. We can't thank her enough.

"I see a lot of unexplained infertility, like James and Christiane's, in my clinic. But what might be unexplained in orthodox medical terms may well have an explanation in Chinese medicine, which looks at more subtle and whole body factors. Infertility is 'unexplained' if a couple has not conceived in a year of trying, and neither partner has been diagnosed with a condition that would affect their fertility. This includes, for women, endometriosis, polycystic ovarian disease, age (older than 38 years), tubal blockage, or autoimmune conditions. For men, infertility is diagnosed by certain parameters measured in a semen analysis that relate to the number of sperm, their shape, how well they swim, and the integrity of their DNA.

"When couples struggle to conceive—for whatever reason—they often feel incredibly frustrated. Sometimes having a label that leads to a definitive treatment is an easier diagnosis to cope with. However, treatments for many of the conditions that lead to infertility do not have simple and straightforward treatments with guaranteed outcomes.

"Whether or not couples can help themselves depends on the cause of their infertility, but generally there is much couples can do to improve their fertility. Let's start with men, because it is often easier to improve sperm than it is eggs. Lifestyle factors make a big difference to the health of sperm, and the good news is that most of it is under your control. Heavy alcohol consumption has a deleterious effect on sperm count and function, but moderate drinking seems to do no harm. All relevant studies have shown the negative effects of tobacco or marijuana on sperm. If you're having difficulty giving up either of these, seek help immediately if you're trying to conceive. As for coffee, a little bit is fine for most men, but more than three cups a day has been shown to damage sperm DNA. Being overweight is associated with decreased testosterone and increased estrogen, neither of which is good news for your sperm count or quality. Now is a good time to start a weight-loss program. Acupuncture can help control your appetite and accelerate weight loss.

"Frequent sex improves the quality of sperm, while a few days' abstinence increases the quantity of sperm. So when the woman is ovulating, daily sex around this time is recommended. If not, have sex every second day from when her period finishes and continue for ten days (or more if she has a long cycle). We also know that men exposed to chemicals or fumes at their workplace have lower sperm counts, so try your best to limit exposure. We know that electromagnetic radiation from mobile phones and laptops is associated with hormone changes and that long hours of use are associated with reduced fertility. Do not keep your mobile phone in the side pocket of your trousers and try to limit its use.

"Lastly, a number of clinical studies have shown the beneficial effects of acupuncture and Chinese herbs in improving sperm quality and fertility. More than ten separate trials in a number of different countries have all shown a significant improvement in sperm morphology and motility after a course of acupuncture.

"For women, the underlying cause (if there is one) needs to be addressed. Endometriosis is usually treated with surgery, and polycystic ovarian disease is often treated with drugs that reduce insulin levels (diabetes drugs) and drugs to induce ovulation if necessary. We don't yet have effective drug treatments for autoimmune conditions, except steroids which may be used in some situations. Chinese medicine offers very good proven treatments for endometriosis and polycystic ovarian disease.

"In my clinic we see couples with infertility and assess them from a Chinese medicine point of view. This means taking a thorough case history and looking at what investigations have been done already. All aspects of the body and mind are taken into account with a focus on the reproductive system, of course. Sometimes it is clear that Chinese medicine will not help improve fertility (for example, if the fallopian tubes are blocked) and we will refer the couple to an IVF clinic if they wish to take that route.

"For most conditions related to infertility, including those that don't have a Western medicine label, a Chinese medicine program can be formulated and we can expect good results. We use Chinese herbs, which are taken twice daily as a tea (a rather strong-tasting tea, but most people get used to it quickly). Acupuncture is done weekly or bi-weekly, in the case of women for 3–6 months. For men we treat once or twice a week, for 1–3 months, and then retest the sperm. Sometimes we work together with the IVF clinic to prepare a couple who have had previous IVF failures, in the hope that their chances are better with subsequent cycles.

Generally there is much couples can do to improve their fertility.

"We probably see as much secondary infertility as we do primary infertility. These couples are particularly frustrated because they know they have achieved pregnancy at least once before. Often the cause is unexplained from a Western medicine point of view, but Chinese medicine will usually find a cause that may be related to factors that have arisen since the first child or previous children—sometimes this is depletion of internal resources or stress which can upset the hormone balance. Sometimes it is related to age. Improving lifestyle factors like stress, sleep patterns, and digestion often helps with this type of infertility.

"I'm so glad I could help James and Christiane, who will share with you my advice—and plenty more from other experts and themselves—in this book. Good luck."
BY JANE LYTTLETON BSc (Hons) NZ, MPhil Lond, Dip TCM Aus, Cert Ac, Cert Herbal Medicine, China

FERTILITY AND STRESS

For years studies have been showing that stress is linked to fertility—which can lead to a vicious cycle of feeling stressed that you're not getting pregnant, then worrying that stress is making the problem worse. People will say things like, "Don't worry about it and it will just happen." They'll then go on to tell you about their friend who went on vacation or who decided to adopt a baby and who then got pregnant immediately because they had "stopped worrying about it."

Although well-meaning, this sort of advice can be very frustrating, and yet the truth is that stress and fertility are inextricably linked, and that's why I've included it here. A few simple lifestyle changes can make a huge difference and improving your diet and regularly getting more sleep is the perfect place to start.

FOODS THAT REDUCE STRESS

✳ **Berries** are full of vitamin C, which allows the body to cope better with stress. They're also full of fiber, which helps to regulate blood-sugar levels (these can fluctuate when we're stressed).

✳ **Green vegetables** – dark green vegetables help replenish our bodies with vitamins in times of stress.

✳ **Turkey** contains an amino acid called L-tryptophan, which releases serotonin (a calming, feel-good hormone) into the body. Eating turkey has a soothing effect on the body and can even help you sleep better.

✳ **Sweet potatoes** will satisfy a carb craving (common during stressful times, because blood-sugar level swings cause us to crave sugar fixes), and also contain more fiber and vitamins than ordinary potatoes.

✳ **Avocados** – all the good fat and potassium they contain can lower your blood pressure (which rises during times of stress).

✳ **Nuts** help boost an immune system weakened by stress, plus they're full of B vitamins which help to lower stress levels.

FOODS THAT INCREASE STRESS

✳ **Coffee** – too much caffeine stresses out your system by constantly flooding your body with the fat-storing hormone cortisol. Stick to one or two cups of organic coffee a day.

✳ **Alcohol** stimulates the adrenal glands—two tiny glands that sit just above our kidneys and pump out the stress hormone adrenaline. Studies have also shown that alcohol reduces fertility in both sexes, so if you're trying to get pregnant, cut right back or, ideally, stop drinking altogether.

✳ **Sweets and sugary snacks** give you a quick burst of energy, but then they cause your blood-sugar levels to crash, leaving you feeling sluggish, stressed, and lacking concentration.

✳ **Processed foods** are full of so much junk that they deplete the levels of vitamins and minerals in your body, leaving you more prone to stress.

✳ **Junk food** – studies show that foods that are high in bad fats (burgers, fries potato chips, etc.) lower your concentration levels and increase your stress levels.

✳ **Salty foods** increase your blood pressure, which makes you more prone to stress. The worst offenders are processed meats like ham, bacon, and others that are full of salt.

SLEEP YOURSELF LESS STRESSED

Sleep (or a lack of it) and stress often go hand in hand. When we're stressed, we find it more difficult to sleep, and when we're tired, we feel more stressed—it's enough to make you need a nap!

I can't stress enough just how important it is to have sufficient sleep—especially if you're trying to get pregnant. Good restorative sleep is as crucial to brain function and health as are oxygen and water. However, many of us think we can get away with skimping on sleep as we pack more and more into our busy lives. Technology doesn't help matters and neither does the current trend for associating being busy with being important.

Many of us these days are working longer hours than ever and traveling more. And while all these things can enrich our lives to some extent, they can also take their toll on our health. One study from the University of Chicago has found that not sleeping enough can mimic aging—put simply, your body ages prematurely if you don't get enough shut-eye.

So—want to know how can you sleep better? Read on.

SLEEP SMARTER...

Turn off your technology
Too many of us are ruining our sleep with technology—and I for one am guilty of this. It's easy to waste a whole evening browsing mindlessly on our iPads, phones, or laptops when we could be exercising, seeing friends, having a conversation with our partner, or relaxing in a nice bath. Technology was designed to save us time, but instead it can rob us of time, leaving us feeling stressed. It can also delay bedtime. Plus, the flickering light from screens stimulates our brains in a way that makes falling asleep afterward more difficult.

Limit the time you spend using technology in the evenings and do something more relaxing instead. If you don't browse on your phone for an hour before bed, your sleep will automatically become deeper and leave you feeling more refreshed in the morning.

Avoid caffeine
This is so obvious I can't believe I'm saying it, but so many of us forget about the sleep-robbing effects of caffeine.

*top tip
Too many of us take our technology to bed. Keep phones, and iPads and laptops out of the bedroom!

Never, ever be tempted by a 4pm latte. No matter how immune you think you are to the effects of caffeine, it will disrupt your sleep. It interferes with the way the body processes the enzyme adenosine that causes us to feel drowsy and fall asleep and so results in wakefulness. Lack of sleep in turn causes you to feel more stressed the next day and, ironically, more likely to rely on caffeine—and so the cycle continues. Remember, it's also found in regular tea, green tea, soft drinks, chocolate, and certain medications (see p. 14).

Add a few drops of lavender oil to your evening bath
You'll fall asleep more easily. There's a reason why sleep experts tell moms to bathe their babies before bed to help them sleep better—soaking in warm water helps us fall into a deeper sleep, according to several studies.

Stick to a routine
Try to go to bed and wake up at approximately the same time every day, even on weekends. Our sleep–wake cycle is regulated by our circadian clock—a type of internal alarm clock that reminds the brain when to release sleep and wake hormones and when not to. Keeping consistent sleep time strengthens this clock, and you'll sleep more soundly as a result.

Don't argue, worry, eat, drink alcohol, or smoke...
You shouldn't be doing either of the latter anyway, if you're trying to conceive, but try not to do any of these too close to bedtime.

Keep your bedroom for sleep and sex
Sex, by the way, promotes better sleep! Orgasm releases the hormone prolactin, which leads to feelings of relaxation and sleepiness and results in a good night's sleep. Furthermore, dopamine and oxytocin are also released and these create a feeling of well-being, which also leads to a restful sleep.

PRE-PREGNANCY EXERCISES TO BOOST FERTILITY

There are specific muscles and movements that you are going to need in order to stay healthy, pain-free, and fully functional throughout your pregnancy. This program is designed to give you a beautiful, strong foundation for a happy, healthy pregnancy.

Perform each exercise once; the whole routine should take you only about ten minutes, and I would like you to do it every day, if possible. The message here—as it is throughout the whole of this book—is to be kind to yourself. Don't overdo exercise, especially if you're trying to get pregnant. Over-exercising can have as much of an impact on fertility as being unfit or overweight. Being underweight and not having enough body fat can affect your menstrual cycle and your ability to become pregnant.

As you do the exercises in this chapter, repeat this little mantra as it will give you something positive to focus on, and I promise it will make you feel better:

"I'm in perfect health, I'm ready for my healthy, beautiful baby, I deserve a happy, healthy life."

If you'd rather not use the mantra, and you think I'm a weirdo, that's fine! Just be sure to do the exercises, because they're great.

Important note: Seek advice from your physician or health professional if you are in any doubt about exercising while trying to conceive.

EXERCISE	REPS	SETS	REST
Tummy vacuum	8–10	1	30 secs
Superman	10–15/side	1	30 secs
Plank	15–30-sec hold	1	30 secs
Push-up from the knees	5	1	30 secs
Y	10–15	1	60 secs

HOW TO PERFORM THE EXERCISES

Perform the following exercises at the beginning of every workout to ensure your lower back, core (see p. 31), and shoulders are activated and engaged and ready for the workout. Perform each exercise in turn, doing the stated number of repetitions and taking the stated amount of rest between each exercise. Once the final exercise is completed, move on to the circuit program on p. 34.

Tummy vacuum

Start position: Support yourself on your hands and knees with hands under shoulders, arms straight and knees under hips. Make sure your arms and thighs remain at right angles to the floor and keep your back straight and your head aligned with your upper back.

The movement: Relax your stomach, letting it sag toward the floor while maintaining a flat back. Then squeeze your tummy muscles and pull your belly button toward the ceiling, still maintaining a flat back and hold for 5 seconds. Repeat 8–10 times.

*top tip
As you draw your belly button toward your spine, squeeze your pelvic-floor muscles (that stop the flow of urine) as this helps prepare for an easier birth and recovery.

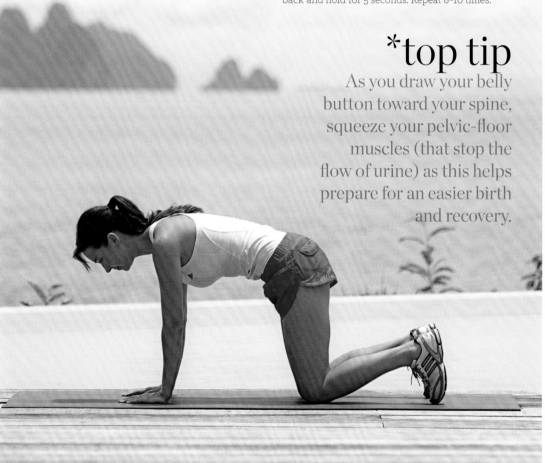

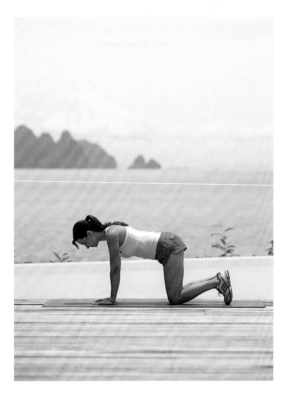
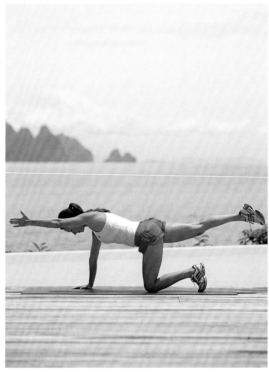

Superman

Start position: Support yourself on your hands and knees with hands under shoulders and knees under hips and with your toes firmly pointed into the floor. Make sure your spine and neck are in a straight line by keeping your gaze to the floor, just in front of your fingertips.

The movement: Extend your left arm out in front of you beyond your head, thumb up, while extending your right leg backward—imagine you are being pulled from either end. Return to the start position and repeat 10–15 times on each side.

*top tip

This exercise will activate and strengthen your hamstrings, glutes, and lower-back muscles, as well as improve your overall body balance.

*top tip

To set the core, pull your belly button in toward the spine so your stomach muscles are engaged.

Plank

Start position: Lie face down on the floor with forearms and elbows touching the floor, hips and legs on the ground.

The movement: Keeping your head aligned with your upper back, raise your hips and set the core. Imagine a straight line from your head to your ankles. Hold for 15–30 seconds, then return to the start position.

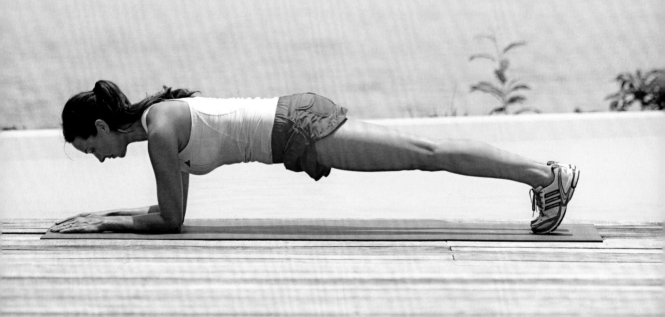

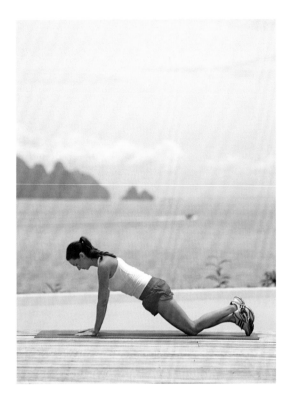
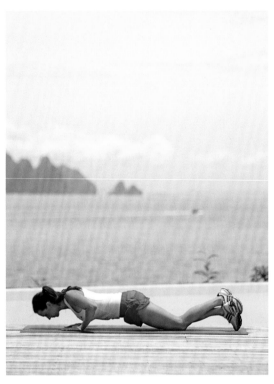

Push-up from the knees

Start position: Place your knees on the ground. Set your hands shoulder-width apart and in line with your nipples, not your shoulders. Keep your ears, shoulders, and hips in alignment and your feet crossed behind you, toes down and pushing into the floor for stability. Set the core by pulling your belly button in toward the spine.

The movement: Keeping your body straight, lower yourself so your nose almost touches the ground, then lift back up to the start position. Remember to ensure that your spine and neck are in a straight line by keeping your gaze to the floor, just in front of your fingertips. Keep your belly button drawn in, then breathe out as you push up to the start position, and breathe in as you lower down. Repeat 5 times.

*top tip

Keep your belly button drawn in to help improve the connection between your brain and your tummy muscles.

If you find this too difficult, start in the same position as above but with your torso elevated with your hands on a chair or couch. The higher up your arms are, or the less horizontal the body is, the easier the push-up will be.

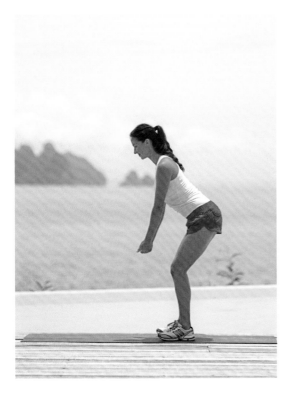

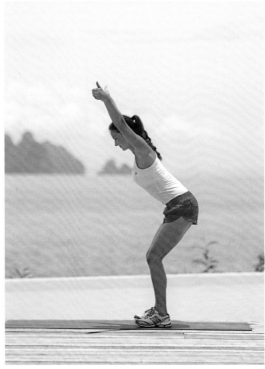

Y

Start position: With your feet hip-width apart, bend your knees and stick your bottom out, so your upper body leans forward 45 degrees. Hold your hands directly below your chest with fists clenched and thumbs up, keeping your head and back in a straight line, your shoulders back and down, and your core tight.

The movement: Raise both hands to create a "Y" shape above your head with your arms by your ears, then return to the starting point. Repeat 10–15 times.

*top tip

Perform this exercise slowly and with control to ensure your body stays relaxed. The less the body is stressed, the easier it can be to become pregnant.

CIRCUIT TRAINING

At Bodyism, we love to get our clients to perform circuits like the one below. This type of circuit is a great way to work lots of muscles and improve your posture, as well as get a great cardiovascular workout without spending time on a bike or treadmill.

The circuit below is designed to strengthen in particular those muscles you're going to need to be robust during the early stages of your pregnancy, as well as post-pregnancy once your beautiful baby is here—your lower back, hamstrings, shoulders, back, and core/tummy muscles. All of these muscle groups need to be strong to help with the added weight gained during pregnancy, as well as to help create a stable, strong body that can handle the birth process. Do each exercise, one after the other, performing the stated number of repetitions and taking the stated amount of rest between each exercise. Once the final exercise is completed, rest for 90 seconds before performing the stated number of sets.

EXERCISE	REPS	SETS	REST
Plié squat	12–15	2–3	30 secs
L to shoulder press	10–12	2–3	30 secs
Flamingo	10–12/ side	2–3	30 secs
Bent-over row (holding ball)	10–12	2–3	30 secs
Side plank	15–30-sec hold/side	2–3	60 secs

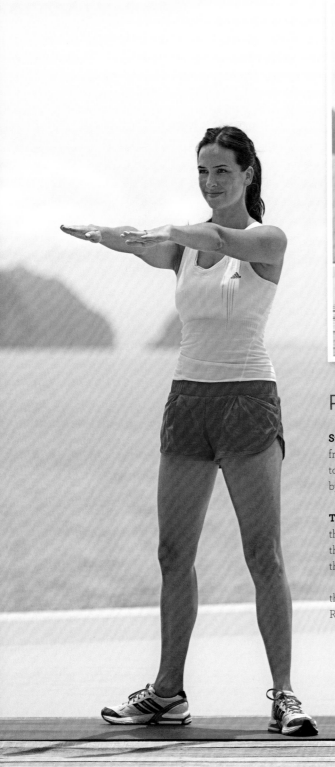

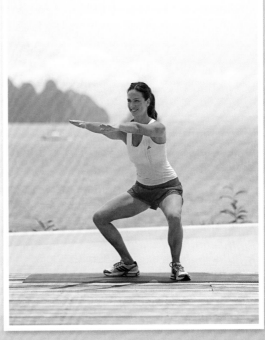

Plié squat

Start position: Stand with your arms straight out in front at shoulder height, feet shoulder-width apart and toes pointed out at 45 degrees. Keep your core engaged by pulling your belly button in toward your spine.

The movement: Keeping your arms straight, initiate the movement by pushing the hips back and bending the knees so you squat back and down until your thighs are parallel to the floor.

Return to the standing position by pushing through the hips and the heels while keeping your torso upright. Repeat 12–15 times.

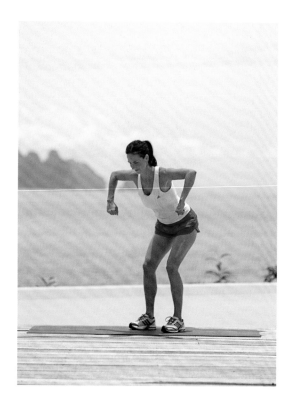

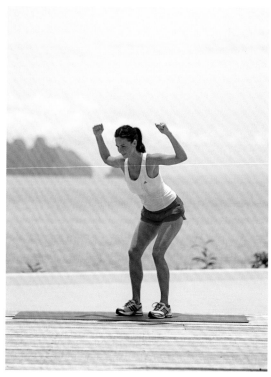

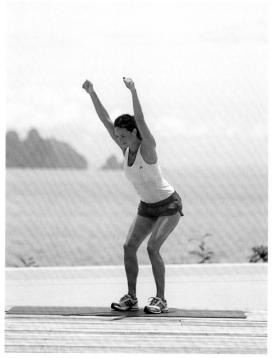

L to shoulder press

Start position: Take a comfortable stance with your feet hip-width apart. Bend your knees and stick your bottom out so your upper body hinges forward from the hips. Keep your head and back in a straight line, shoulders back and down, arms by your sides, palms facing backward. Engage your core by pulling your belly button in toward your spine.

The movement: With your core engaged, bring your arms upward, leading with your elbows until they reach shoulder height. Rotate your forearms upward until the backs of your hands face the ceiling, making an "L" shape with your arms, then straighten your arms upward to perform a shoulder-press movement. Reverse this pattern back to the starting position and repeat 10–12 times.

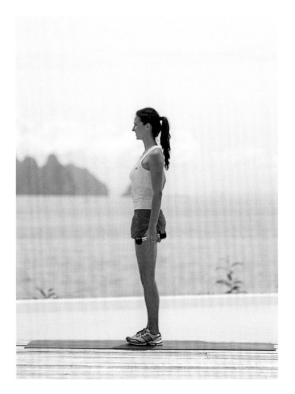
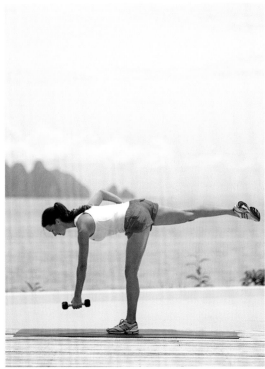

Flamingo

Start position: Stand with your feet together, right hand on your waist and the left holding a light weight by your side. Keep your core engaged by pulling your belly button in toward your spine.

The movement: Hinge over at your waist by pushing your right leg back behind you. Allow the arm holding the weight to lower as shown. Be sure to keep your standing leg slightly bent, while your back and neck remain in a perfect line. Return to the start position and repeat 10–12 times on each side.

*top tip
This exercise is great for strengthening your hamstrings. Perform it slowly and with control to create stability in the lower body.

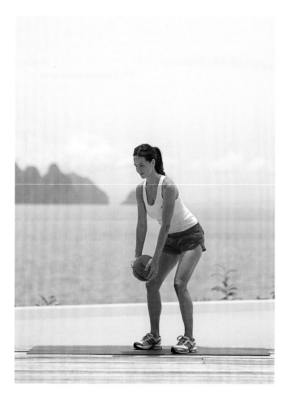

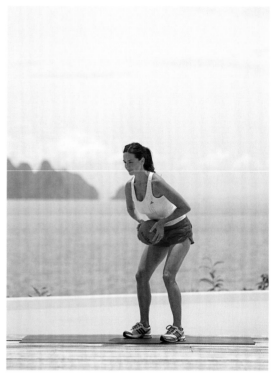

Bent-over row
(holding ball)

Start position: Stand with feet shoulder-width apart and, holding either a ball or dumbbell, hinge over at the waist. Make sure your neck and spine are in a straight line by fixing your gaze slightly down and in front of you and engage your core by pulling your belly button in toward the spine.

The movement: Slide your shoulder blades back and pull your elbows toward the sky, raising the ball or dumbbell up to your belly button. Lower the ball/dumbbell back down to the start position and repeat 10-12 times.

*top tip

This exercise targets the postural muscles in the back. Good postural alignment not only strengthens the skeletal system but also supports the body's vital organs, including the reproductive organs.

*top tip

Strong and stable core muscles can help prevent back problems during pregnancy and help toward an easier labor and quicker postpartum recovery.

Side plank

Start position: Lie on your side with your feet stacked on top of each other, your right forearm on the ground, your right elbow under your right shoulder and your left hand resting on your waist. Engage your core by pulling your belly button in toward the spine.

The movement: Keeping your elbow under your shoulder and your legs straight, lift your hips into the air so that there is a straight line from the top of your head to your heel. Keep your core engaged and hold for 15–30 seconds, then repeat on the opposite side.

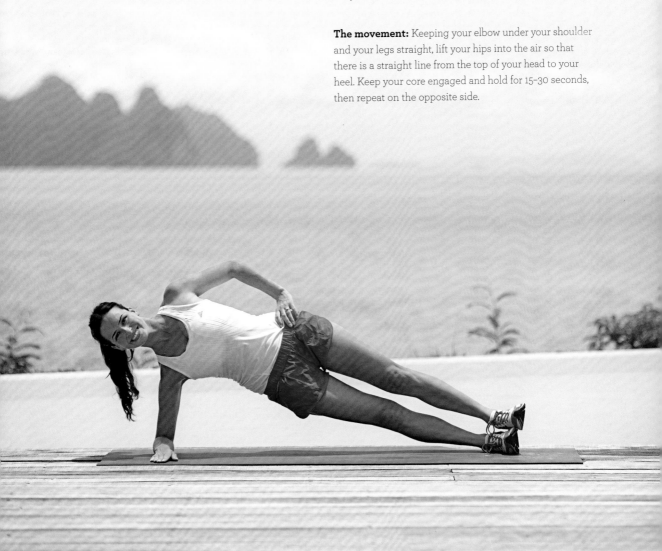

SALLY OBERMEDER

"For me, being pregnant was the most amazing experience I have ever had! To know that a precious being was growing inside me with my help just made me feel so lucky and it had extra special meaning as it had taken me so long to decide when the exact right time was to have a baby and then to get pregnant. Naively, I thought that as soon as I had decided to have a baby, that it would happen immediately. For the other big hurdles of my life—a career change and major weight loss—there was a direct correlation between effort and result, so I thought baby-making would be the same. However, after years of trying and struggling and never producing a baby, I realized that this was one of those life events that plays by a different set of rules. In the end I found success with IVF, and very fortunately after just one cycle.

"I was a little apprehensive about what my pregnancy would be like. I don't know if I was insanely lucky or just stuck floating on cloud nine, but I had no bad experiences at all—well, my boobs got huge, but I guess that's not something to complain about! No morning sickness, no weird cravings for pickles dipped in peanut butter, or hot dog hankerings at 2am. I wanted to be as healthy as I could be for myself and my much-longed-for baby. I kept up my fitness routine, adapting it to my ever-growing belly; I started Pilates classes and I truly have never felt healthier, happier, or more content. I know everyone says this about their babies but she was my little miracle and already she had my spirit—even though she needed a little nudge through IVF to get here, she was a fighter and stubborn and she was going to get here one way or another.

"At the very end of my pregnancy and ironically when I was feeling my best, I was hit with the very hardest blow I have ever had. The day before Annabelle was born, I was diagnosed with stage 3 breast cancer. The cancer was both rare and aggressive and the outlook was not at all good. I knew then and there that I had no choice but to fight like a warrior and make it through for my baby. We had gone through so much to get here and I couldn't let our relationship end before it had even begun.

"Chemo was tough, so tough that there were days when I really did just want to give up—to this day I don't really know exactly what it did to my husband Marcus, who was of course so worried about losing me, and yet he was always there as my rock and helping me through some of the most harrowing moments.

"And then there was Annabelle. I had so much I wanted to share with my daughter and there was no way I was going to let her grow up without a mother. Sometimes I still grieve for my first year of motherhood—it wasn't at all how I thought it would be. No play groups or play dates with other mothers, just chemo and scans, tests and radiation, surgery, and more surgery. I felt guilty that I wasn't being a 'proper' mom to Annabelle but I would remind myself that I was fighting this fight with every ounce of the limited physical strength that I had, just to ensure that I would live to see her first steps, first words, her first day at school and all the firsts that every parent longs to witness.

"I am incredibly blessed to still be here today and am the happiest I've ever been. I know it's an overused phrase, but I've learned to savor every moment, to be 'in the moment.' I close my eyes and take pictures with my memory and soak up every detail. I'm proud to say I have a happy, healthy 2-year-old monkey, a loving husband, and amazing family and friends. I may have scars all over my body as a result of the many surgeries, but I'm proud of them and every time I look at Annabelle I think how far we've come together."

> *She was my little miracle and already she had my spirit—she was a fighter and stubborn and she was going to get here one way or another.*

YOGA FOR FERTILITY

Yoga has completely changed our lives. It is difficult to express how grateful Christiane and I are to the yoga experts Wenche Beard, Una Laffan, and Danai Kougiouli who gave us love and support while we were trying to get pregnant and every moment since then, and who have contributed incredible routines for this book.

Una is an amazing lady. She has studied Ashtanga Vinyasa Yoga and other forms of movement and dance therapies in Mexico, the US, and India and I'm so happy she is able to share her wisdom here:

"In the pre-conception stage we need to be gentle with ourselves and our bodies. Enjoy a yoga practice that nourishes and soothes your system and allows you to find space where you can slow down and ground yourself. The following sequence emphasizes breath, softness, and openness. It focuses on the hips and pelvis to improve the flow of energy through these parts of your body. The connection between your breath and movement will calm the mind and help you feel in touch, in tune, and in love with your body. The routine is designed as a fluid progression so perform each pose and then move on to the next."

BY UNA LAFFAN

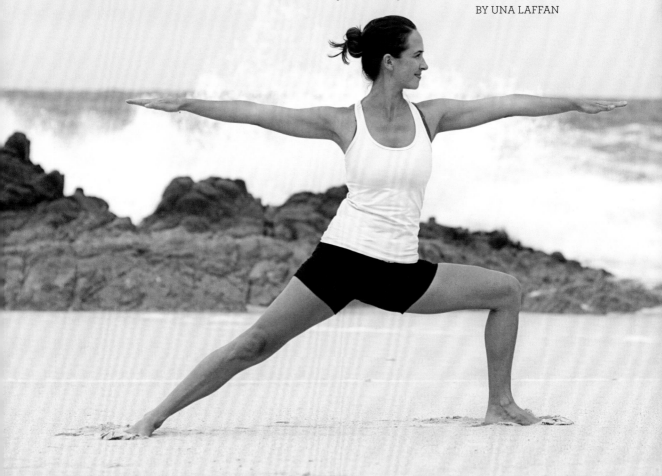

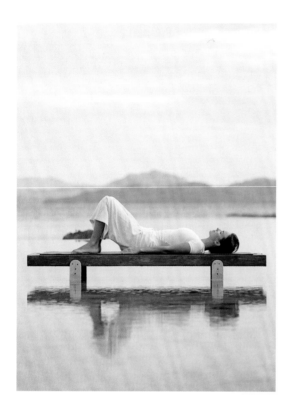
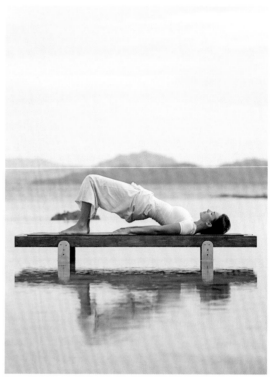

Setu Bandhasana (Supported bridge pose)

Lie on your back, knees raised, with feet hip-width apart, toes and thighs parallel, heels close to your sitting bones. Take a moment to find your breath and feel your breath soften your stomach, chest, throat, and face.

As you exhale, press your feet into the earth and let your hips lift up, lengthening your tailbone toward the knees and keeping your thighs and inner feet parallel.

Without squeezing the buttocks, allow the strength of your legs and feet to support your hips and keep the breath soft into the belly. Relax your internal organs. Enjoy the opening and softening of your belly and chest area as you feel the strength and support of your legs, back, and shoulders. Breathe a few rounds of breath as you connect your feet into the earth, then come down for 2 breaths. Repeat 3–4 times.

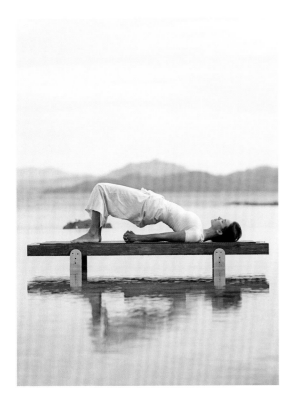

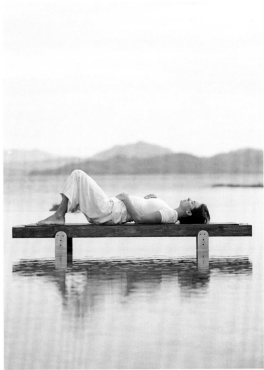

A deeper variation: When your hips are raised, interlace your hands underneath your back on the floor. Be gentle and breathe here for at least 5 breaths, as your front body softens into the support of your lower and back body. Repeat 3–4 times.

To finish, lower your hips slowly to the ground, relaxing your spine down. Take a moment to rest with one palm on your lower belly and the other on your heart. Feel the breath under your palms as you soften your jaw, heart, and belly. Rest and delight in your breath until you feel your body is ready to move on.

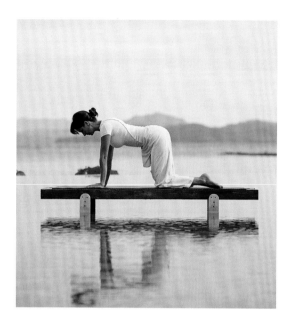

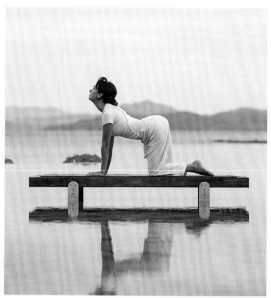

Marjaryasana/Bitilasana (Cat pose/Cow pose)

Start in a "table-top" position with your palms under your shoulders and your knees directly under your hips and your neck in line with your torso.

As you inhale, open your belly to the earth; pointing your tailbone to the sky, open your chest through your arms and lengthen the back of your neck as you softly look up. Feel the openness of your front body.

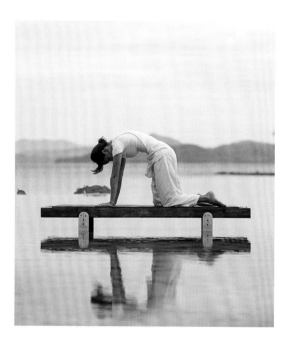

As you exhale, press your hands and knees into the floor and curl up into your chest, sternum, and belly. Opening your back ribs to the sky, relax your head and hips down. Repeat the movement between these two poses 5 times, moving and breathing slowly so you can enjoy the transitions.

*top tip

These movements provide a gentle massage to the spine and belly organs and they help ease the back torso and neck. They are also beneficial for releasing stress.

Balasana
(Child's pose)

From table-top position, move into Child's Pose with your hips over your heels, arms lengthened out in front of you, forehead resting on the floor (or a cushion) and your neck and arms relaxed. Rest for 5–10 breaths.

Slide forward, back into table-top position, before moving gradually into standing.

*top tip

This pose calms the brain and helps relieve stress and fatigue. It also helps open the hips, thighs and ankles.

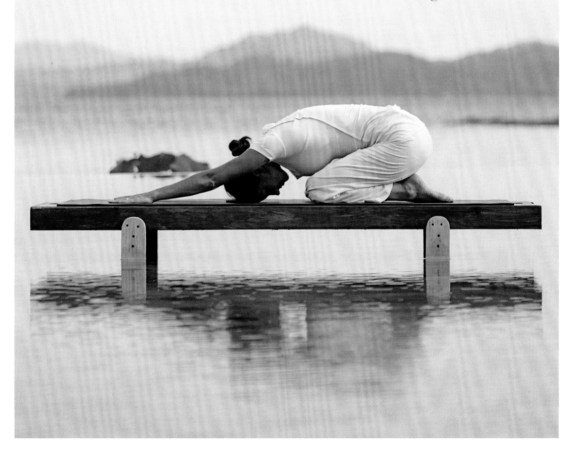

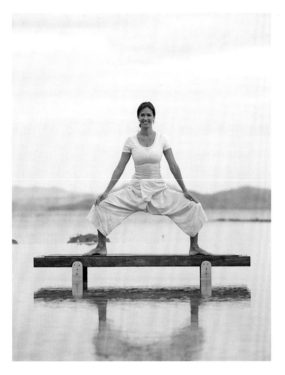

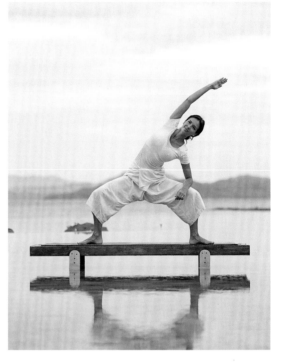

Utkata Konasana (Goddess pose)

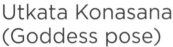

Stand with feet a little wider than hip-width apart and toes open at a 45-degree angle, knees bent in the direction of your middle toe, thighs rotated outward, spine relaxed, and tailbone pointing to the floor. Rest your hands on your thighs and soften your shoulders and upper body into the strength of your legs. Breathe evenly and softly for 5 breaths. (You may straighten your legs for a rest.)

Come back to your squat and, as you inhale, place the left elbow onto your left thigh (or place your hand, if this feels like too much). Exhale and lengthen from your right hip into your right ribs, as you open your right arm over your ear and over your head, your side opening to the sky. Breathe in this pose for 5 breaths.

Inhale back into the center with a neutral spine and exhale, then repeat on the other side. Do this 3 times, then return to standing to rest your legs before the next pose.

*top tip
This pose strengthens and stretches the thighs, hips, groin, knees, and ankles and it helps increase circulation in these areas. Side-opening helps open the waist, chest, lungs, and shoulders and stimulates the abdominal organs.

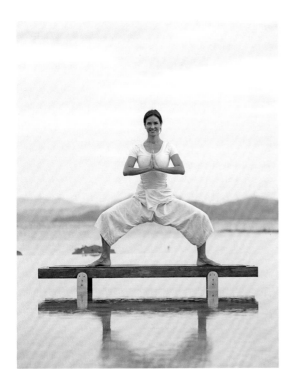

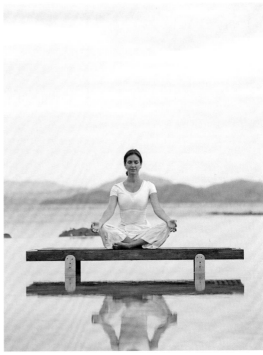

Inhale and come back to the center in your squat, placing both palms together in front of your heart. This hand gesture is used to induce a meditative state of awareness. It is also a gesture to express reverence, honor, and celebration.

As you remain in this pose, breathe into your lower body. Allow a little intensity and heat to arise in your thighs and legs. Feel the reverence in your heart, honor your body, and celebrate in your heart as you welcome life (and flow) into your body and pelvis.

You can hold this pose for up to 3 minutes, but start with 1 minute and build up slowly.

At the end of your practice, come to a comfortable seated position. You can raise your hips on a cushion or a bolster and cross your feet in front of you.

Rest your hands on your legs or knees and let your index finger and thumb touch. Close your eyes and receive your breath with your belly and relax your pelvic floor as you inhale. Soften and surrender as you exhale, and release your breath and anything that it would serve you to let go of. Feel free to lie down on your back with your palms open by your sides.

*top tip
This pose increases stamina and the circulation of energy.

TOP TEN FOODS TO BOOST FERTILITY

Here are ten Clean & Lean foods that will help to improve and extend not only your fertility, but also that of your partner. If you're already pregnant or a mom, eat them anyway to keep you healthy and feeling great.

FOR HER...

1. Full-fat dairy: Researchers from Harvard University found women who eat at least one serving of full-fat dairy a day reduce their risk of infertility by more than a quarter. The dairy is thought to help improve ovarian function. Forget low-fat or diet yogurts as they often contain sugar to make up for the lack of fat. Instead, dive into full-fat Greek yogurt, organic milk, and quality (less-processed) cheese.

2. Olive oil: Harvard researchers found that olive and certain other oils—like flaxseed—can boost female fertility by promoting proper hormone function.

3. Folate-rich foods: Folic acid, also known as vitamin B₉, is essential for all women who are trying to conceive or in the first 12 weeks of pregnancy as it protects against neural tube defects such as spina bifida. A 400mcg supplement is recommended, together with folate-rich foods such as broccoli, spinach, asparagus, and lentils.

4. Orange fruit and vegetables: The body converts orange foods that are rich in beta-carotene to vitamin A, which supports healthy ovulation.

5. Vegetarian protein: According to a study at Harvard University, women who eat more plant proteins (e.g. nuts, chickpeas, and legumes), are more likely to get pregnant than those who get their proteins from red meat as the latter are harder to digest and this can send hormone levels out of balance, thus affecting fertility.

6. Oily fish: The omega-3 fatty acids found in oily fish help to regulate reproductive hormones, relieve stress, and increase blood flow to the sexual organs. Vegetarians can get omega-3 fatty acids from walnuts, pumpkin seeds, flaxseed oil, and eggs.

FOR HIM...

1. Spinach: It's a great source of folate, which improves sperm production. A study from the University of California found that men who regularly eat spinach had up to 30 percent healthier sperm, so eat it a couple of times a week to improve your fertility.

2. Honey: Researchers at the University of Western Australia found that the antioxidants present in honey may prevent sperm damage and increase sperm health. Pick a good-quality manuka honey, as it contains more health-boosting antioxidants than regular honey. Spread it thinly on whole-grain flatbreads or fresh rye bread.

3. Brazil nuts: A study from the University of Padua showed that just three of these a day can prevent damage to sperm from environmental factors.

4. Brightly colored fruits and vegetables: Researchers at the University of Rochester, NY found that brightly colored fruits and vegetables such as tomatoes, beets, bell peppers, and oranges, which contain the antioxidants glutathione and cryptoxanthin, are associated with strong, healthy sperm.

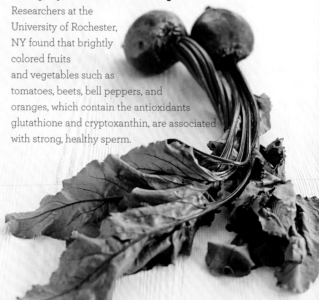

OUR COVER GIRL'S STORY

My wife Christiane gave birth to our beautiful daughter Charlotte in 2012. Here's her story.

"Being a mom is even more amazing than I ever expected. Every moment with Charlotte is heart-warming and it often feels like she's been in our lives forever. I now know what it feels like to be completely fulfilled and content. But the road to getting pregnant was long and rocky, so we know first-hand how difficult fertility struggles can be.

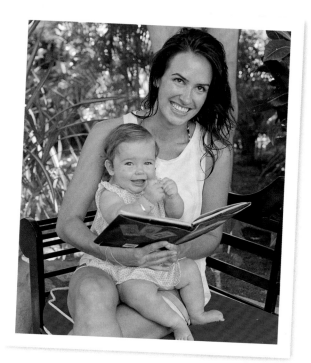

"After a wonderful wedding in the summer of 2010 James and I started trying for a family immediately. As you'd expect, we're both fit and healthy; James has spent his whole career getting people into shape, and he's advised lots of female clients who were trying to conceive. So, if I'm being honest, I took our fertility for granted.

"Coming from a family of healthy, fertile women I never thought I'd have any issues myself. But after James and I got married I had my contraceptive implant removed, and my period never arrived. I chalked it up to my body adjusting and the fact that I traveled a lot for work. But as the months went by and I still wasn't pregnant, we started to worry.

"After what felt like the longest year of my life, we saw a specialist who told us, following various tests, that there was no medical reason for our inability to conceive. It wasn't a relief—it was just incredibly frustrating. At least if there was a problem we could try to fix it, but all we could do was live in an awful state of limbo and keep on hoping.

"We're positive people, but the sadness started to set in. I looked at our friends and family and everybody around us seemed to be having babies. When would it be our turn? It wasn't fair and we felt utterly powerless. I remember sitting in our gynecologist's office in tears as he explained that we might never conceive.

"But I knew in my heart that my purpose in life was to have lots of children, so I never gave in to the negative results and comments. I wanted to take some control over the situation, so with the advice of fertility experts I tweaked my diet, which was good anyway. I cut down on the amount I was exercising. (Too much exercise,

especially cardio, can put extra stress on the body and make your cycles irregular; it was making me underweight, too.) I also turned to alternative therapies like acupuncture and reflexology.

"James and I stayed positive and I kept telling myself it would happen. I still knew I was destined to be a mother, and I couldn't see a future without a child in it, so I trusted that it would happen at the right time.

"We were offered fertility-enhancing drugs, but we wanted to take a more natural route. However, as the months went on, we eventually decided to try Clomid, which is used to induce ovulation. Amazingly, though, my period arrived the day we were due to get the drug.

"Still the months went on and I wasn't pregnant. It was incredibly hard, but we used to repeat these little mantras to each other every day about how grateful we were for having each other, our friends, family, and soon our little healthy baby. We decided we didn't want this struggle to make us bitter or angry. I'm not saying that it was always easy or that we never felt those emotions, but it helped us.

"Then a chance meeting with an old friend and her daughter led us to consider IVF. It's important for me to mention that we'd never had anything against IVF; we had just decided it wasn't for us at the start. But after seeing our friend's utterly beautiful baby we realized we had to go for it.

"We booked an appointment for IVF, but another coincidence was around the corner: on the day of our appointment, I had a really weird feeling I was pregnant. Although my periods had returned, I was now a week late. Initially I had just put this down to my cycle being irregular, but that morning I took a pregnancy test and watched wide-eyed as the line appeared to show it was positive. Despite the fact that this was everything I'd ever dreamed of, I didn't jump for joy. I felt calm and almost detached and, looking back, I guess I didn't want to get my hopes up in case it wasn't true. I showed James the test and he was also very calm. We had a cuddle with big smiles and teary eyes and both felt quietly happy, hoping and praying this was it and that we'd finally get our baby.

"As the pregnancy progressed, I let myself relax and then I became really excited as I watched my bump grow. However, I had terrible morning sickness. I desperately wanted to eat healthily for the baby, but I was vomiting the whole time and just craved white carbs (in Chapter 8 James gives plenty of tips on dealing with cravings in a Clean & Lean way). I soon learned that my baby would take everything it needed from me to be healthy and leave me without! So I kept my vitamin supply up with a prenatal multivitamin. My energy levels were very low and I would find myself in bed all day. I was putting on weight and watching my belly grow and, as beautiful as this process is, I started feeling bad about myself. This was not what I was expecting. I had to turn these feelings around because my baby and I were now one. Anything I felt, the baby would also feel.

"I made a point of still going for walks and doing gentle yoga as this helped keep me feeling good and strong. I learned to listen to my body and do what it told me, but taking away any shame or guilt about myself or what I was doing. I learned to embrace the entire process and all the beautiful changes that my body was going through, so that my baby would grow healthy and strong inside me. One of the first of many sacrifices we make for our children! But the end result, having that baby safely in your arms, is a blissful feeling that is indescribable.

"Thankfully, my labor was straightforward and Charlotte was born weighing seven pounds. It was a drug-free, natural labor with only James and the midwife in the room with me. I had done a lot of preparation for it which made me feel empowered and excited about the birth. I had visualized exactly how I wanted it to go and it went to plan. And then came Charlotte; I felt completely overwhelmed when they put her on my chest. I took in her tiny features and couldn't believe she was here at last, as I always knew she would be.

Now every time we look at Charlotte we are so grateful. We would have waited a lifetime for her to come into our lives.

"Life since Charlotte's birth has been so wonderful, full of joy, love, and peace. James is the most amazing, loving and supportive father and the best thing of all is that he is always there. Times are not always easy with a newborn—there is so much to learn for both mom and baby. There are many nights with broken sleep, cries when you just wish you could take away their distress, an extraordinary amount of hormones flooding through your body, and energy-zapping breastfeeding.

"What really worked for us was having a routine from day one. It helps us to predict why Charlotte may be crying, and to know that she is getting enough sleep and food. All her needs are being met now, as well as mine. And when we put Charlotte to bed at 7pm and James and I have the evening to ourselves, all we do is look at pictures and watch videos of her from the day!

"I now look back on my journey and in a way I feel grateful it took so long because I now know what it means to be truly healthy. It's about eating well and mindfully (and now passing this on to Charlotte while weaning her), doing balanced exercise, using natural therapies, learning to relax through meditation, trusting in life and my body, and keeping a strong and positive mind, free from shame and guilt."

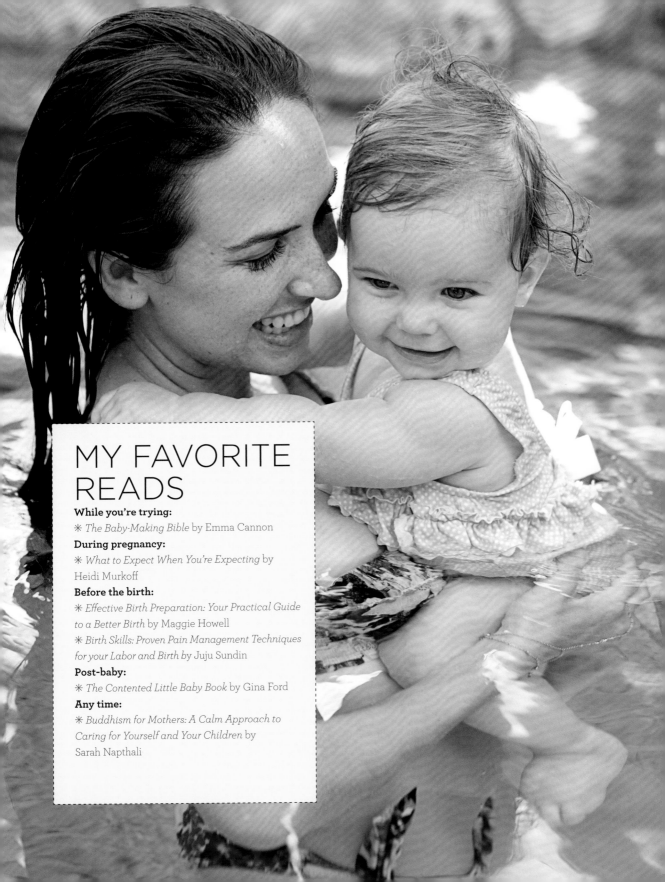

MY FAVORITE READS

While you're trying:
✻ *The Baby-Making Bible* by Emma Cannon

During pregnancy:
✻ *What to Expect When You're Expecting* by Heidi Murkoff

Before the birth:
✻ *Effective Birth Preparation: Your Practical Guide to a Better Birth* by Maggie Howell
✻ *Birth Skills: Proven Pain Management Techniques for your Labor and Birth* by Juju Sundin

Post-baby:
✻ *The Contented Little Baby Book* by Gina Ford

Any time:
✻ *Buddhism for Mothers: A Calm Approach to Caring for Yourself and Your Children* by Sarah Napthali

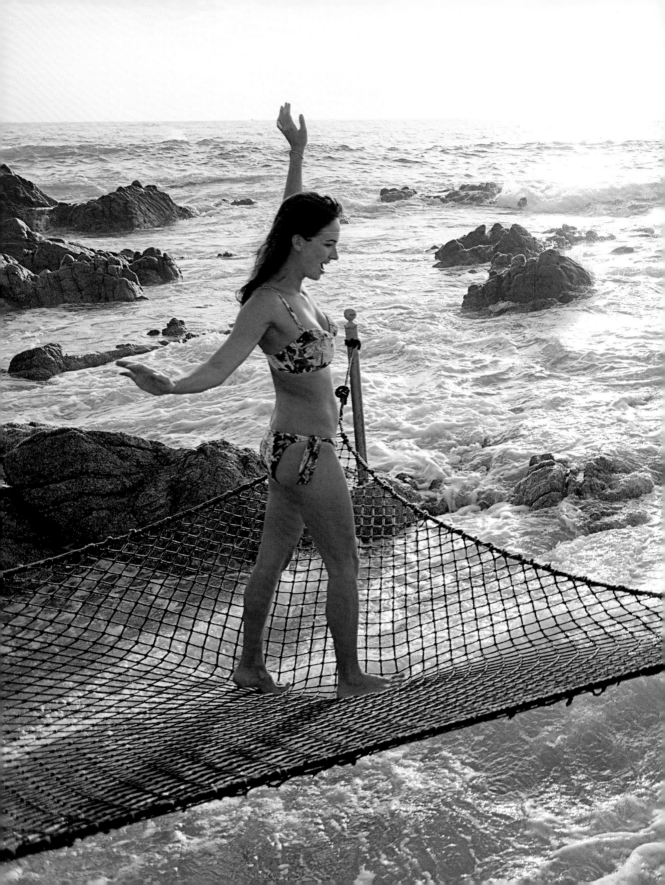

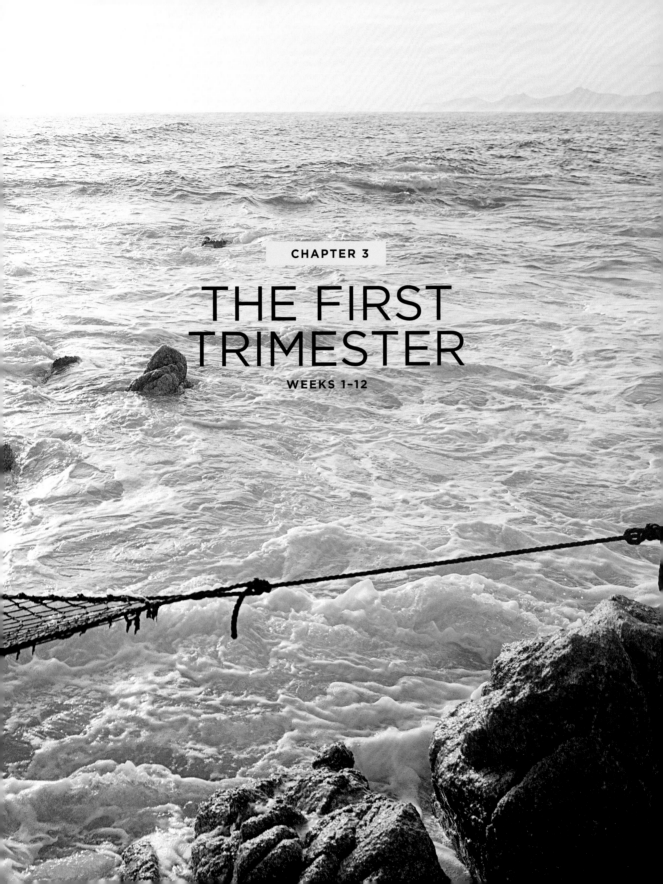

CHAPTER 3

THE FIRST TRIMESTER

WEEKS 1–12

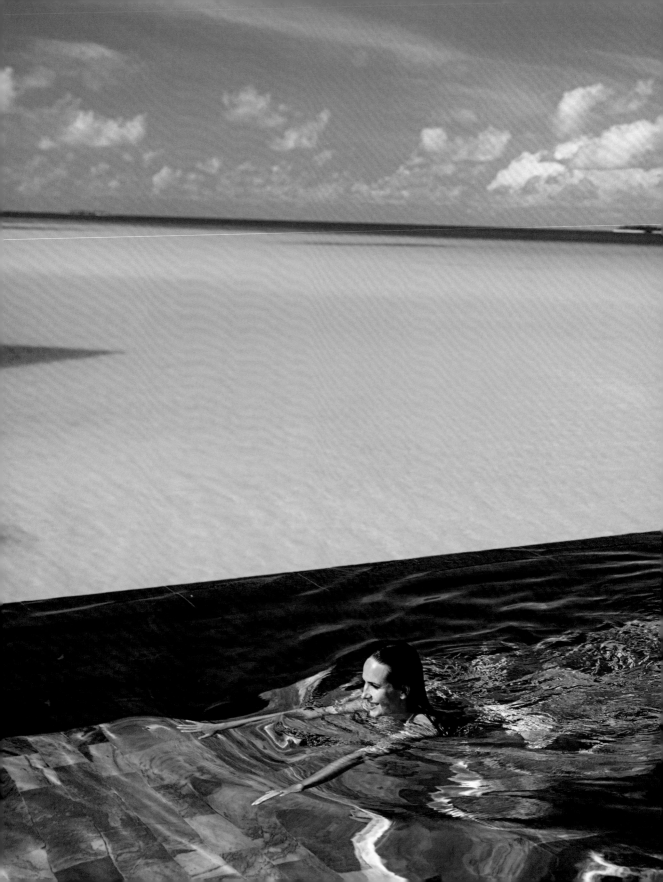

FROM THE MIDWIFE

Having a good midwife to help you through pregnancy is absolutely essential and Christiane and myself were lucky to be supported by the very best—Julie Schiller. Below, she lets you know how your baby is growing in the first trimester.

"At four weeks old, your unborn baby is a cluster of developing cells around the size of a poppy seed. The yolk sac is producing nutrients and red blood cells for your baby, and the placenta and umbilical cord are getting ready to take over. By five weeks, your baby's heart starts to beat, buds are starting to sprout that will eventually become its arms and legs, and organs are beginning to develop. The head is still disproportionately large compared to the body and by nine weeks the genitals are starting to form, although it'll be hard to determine the sex for a few more weeks. By ten weeks all the important organs—such as the brain, lungs, and kidneys—are fully formed. By the end of the first trimester your baby is the size of a lime and can close its fingers and curl its toes. Your uterus, which started off the size of an orange, is now the size of a grapefruit. Much of your baby's crucial development has taken place this trimester and now it's time for it to get bigger and stronger."

BY JULIE SCHILLER

*top tip

Listen to your body during pregnancy. Sit down and rest when your body tells you to and, if you're tired, choose sleep over exercise in this trimester.

The first trimester is often the hardest and most tiring for many women. In fact, one of the first symptoms of pregnancy for some is extreme tiredness. Nobody knows for sure why this is, but it's thought to be due to the hormonal changes that are taking place—especially the increase in the hormones progesterone and estrogen.

The most important thing to do during these first twelve weeks of pregnancy is to listen to your body: so rest when you feel like it, and sleep whenever you can (if this is your first pregnancy, it may be the last chance you'll get for a while); and if you're hungry, eat something. It's that simple. Your body has the amazing ability to tell you exactly what it needs (so listen up), and this is truer now than ever. Nature will always do its job and help your baby grow strong and healthy, so try to relax and embrace all the changes that are coming your way.

That said, you can always tweak your lifestyle to make the first twelve weeks a little easier by eating Clean & Lean. It's one of the best things you can do for yourself and your baby, as you'll both be getting lots of great nutrients and avoiding empty calories and unhealthy additives and toxins. It won't always be easy in the first trimester, when you may be feeling unusually tired, hungry, or sick, so try not to put too much pressure on yourself. If you follow the basics of Clean & Lean 80 percent of the time, it won't matter if you go off track a little. Just remember, as always, to be kind to yourself.

In this chapter I'm going to give you tips and advice on staying Clean & Lean during the first trimester, along with some gentle exercises you can do if you feel up to it. They're not designed to keep you in shape (although that will be an added bonus), but to keep your body strong and supple to carry you through your pregnancy journey. And just a little reminder—you're amazing for creating another little person!

WHAT YOU MAY BE EXPERIENCING RIGHT NOW

Morning sickness

This can often be one of the worst first-trimester symptoms and it affects three quarters of pregnant women. Despite its name, it can occur at any time of the day (or even all day). However, most women experience it in the first half of the day—most likely because they haven't eaten overnight (while they've slept). Experts agree that hormonal changes are the cause of morning sickness.

What to do: One of the best ways to combat it is to keep your blood-sugar levels steady and you can do this by eating Clean & Lean. Eat five small meals a day, which roughly translates as three meals plus a couple of snacks in between. However, keep your meals smaller and your snacks bigger than usual so all five "meals" are approximately the same size.

If you're craving carbohydrates, go for energy-boosting ones like oats, spelt, brown rice, and quinoa. If you crave sugar, have some, but don't go overboard. Sugary foods actually make you more tired in the long run—they give you a hit of energy when you eat them because they cause a massive spike in your blood-sugar levels, but this is followed by a crash, which leaves you tired and craving more sugar. Instead, eat Clean & Lean foods, little and often, and keep treats for the odd occasion when you really crave them.

Swollen, tender breasts

Hormonal surges in the first trimester can make your breasts feel swollen and tender. It isn't milk, which comes along just before you give birth and in the days afterwards.

What to do: This usually settles down after the second trimester but it's a good idea to go for a bra fitting in your first trimester to make sure you're wearing the right size.

TIPS FOR MORNING SICKNESS

✳ Keep a supply of rice cakes by your bed, so if you wake up hungry in the night or first thing in the morning you can munch on them.

✳ Avoid drinking fluids for fifteen minutes before and after meals, and never during mealtimes. Your digestion slows down in pregnancy and drinking fluids slows it down even further. So stay hydrated (see p. 61), but avoid drinking too close to mealtimes.

✳ Don't overdo it—sleep when you're tired, and this will really help with the sickness.

✳ Try ginger—have a cup of ginger tea (see p. 18) or use it ground in your food.

✳ Minimize stress—easier said than done, but try to avoid stressful situations as it's thought stress makes nausea worse.

✳ Try acupuncture or reflexology—find pregnancy-specific experts local to you.

✳ If, despite all of the above, you cannot stop the nausea or losing weight, there are safe medications available. Consult with your midwife or obstetrician.

Excess saliva

Excess saliva in early pregnancy is called ptyalism and it's completely harmless for you and your baby. Doctors don't really know what causes it although, like many pregnancy symptoms, it's thought to be due to changing hormones. **What to do:** Brush your teeth regularly, drink plenty of water, eat small and frequent meals, and avoid starchy foods like bread and potatoes.

Frequent need to urinate

This is another of the first symptoms for many women and it usually starts at around six weeks after conception (and often gets more pronounced with each pregnancy). You can blame your hormones again—they cause more blood flow to your kidneys, so your bladder fills up more quickly. The amount of blood flow in your body rises throughout your pregnancy too, meaning your kidneys also have to process more fluid. Then, as your baby grows, it starts to put more pressure on your bladder. Don't worry, though—apart from being annoying, it's perfectly harmless. **What to do:** Don't be tempted to drink less to avoid too many bathroom trips, as it's important to stay hydrated (in a nutshell, this ensures nutrients from your food are delivered to your baby). However, as long as you've drunk enough in the day it's fine to cut back on water before bedtime to avoid nocturnal bathroom visits. Avoid or cut down on diuretics like tea and coffee, and make sure you fully empty your bladder each time you pee by leaning slightly forward toward the end. Lastly, don't try to hold it in or delay bathroom trips, as this makes the problem worse and could even lead to a UTI (urinary tract infection).

Bleeding gums

The hormone progesterone increases blood flow to the gums, so you may notice you get bleeding gums, especially after brushing your teeth. **What to do:** This should rectify itself after you give birth, but in the meantime brush and floss regularly and gently. If it gets particularly bad, you should see a dentist.

Bloating and gas

Blame those hormones again. Progesterone relaxes the tissue in your gastrointestinal tract, which slows down your digestion, causing gas and bloating. **What to do:** Eat little and often, chew your food

thoroughly (at least fifteen times per mouthful), and try not to drink during meals. And have a sense of humor about it—Christiane and I found the huge truck-driver farts hilarious (she'll love me for telling you that).

Leg cramps

Your already-growing uterus can put pressure on one of the main veins from your legs, creating circulation problems. As you gain weight during pregnancy, the pressure gets worse. Leg cramps can also indicate a nutrient deficiency, such as calcium or magnesium. **What to do:** Drink plenty of fluids and avoid sitting or standing up for long periods. Do simple exercises such as rotating your foot and stretching your calves.

Constipation

Like bloating and gas, this is due to hormonal changes slowing down the digestive tract. It can feel particularly uncomfortable when your baby gets bigger. **What to do:** Drink plenty of water and eat fiber-rich foods, which will also keep your bowels healthy and regular (so helping to prevent hemorrhoids). Gentle exercise helps too, as does a glass of warm water (boil it and wait for it to cool down) with a slice of lemon first thing in the morning to flush out your system.

Food aversions and cravings

Have you suddenly stopped wanting your favorite foods? You're not alone—85 percent of women experience food aversions in early pregnancy. As for cravings, they're often your body's way of telling you what it needs. **What to do:** Many women are turned off by meat protein, so if this is you, try to include some vegetarian protein in your diet instead in the form of beans and pulses (do I hear someone say gas?). Don't worry too much—food aversions usually go away by the second trimester and there are tips for handling cravings in Chapter 8.

Reflux and heartburn

In pregnancy, the hormone progesterone relaxes the valve that separates the esophagus (gullet) and the stomach and this allows stomach acid to come up, causing an uncomfortable burning sensation in the back of the throat. It's made worse by the fact that your digestion is slower and increases as the baby grows and pushes your stomach upwards, shortening your esophagus.

What to do: Avoid carbonated drinks and alcohol, caffeine, sugary, fatty, or spicy foods and citrus fruits. Don't eat big meals—eat several small ones instead (and not too close to bedtime)—and chew thoroughly. Wear loose clothes that aren't tight around your chest, ribcage, or stomach. At night, when it's often worse, prop yourself up using pillows and speak to your doctor or midwife if it's particularly bad as they may prescribe medication.

Irritability

Did you expect you'd feel on top of the world, but find instead that every little thing is annoying you? Don't worry, it's perfectly normal and all down to fluctuating hormones. I just want to share a funny story about Christiane here: when she was expecting Charlotte, she told me off for breathing in an annoying way. I asked her if perhaps her hormones were making her grumpy, and she said: "No, you've just become more annoying since I became pregnant." We laugh about it now, but I'm pretty sure she meant it at the time.

What to do: Try to talk about your concerns to your partner, friends, family, or midwife. Find ways to relax, such as meditation, which will also boost your mood. And if you do feel particularly low and are crying most days, see your doctor or midwife, as it could be a sign of depression.

Dry or spotty skin

Some women find their skin gets drier, more oily, or spotty. And yes—it's those pregnancy hormones yet again.

What to do: Eat Clean & Lean with plenty of skin-loving foods like salmon, vegetables, fruits, and nuts. Cleanse your skin thoroughly (though gently) and drink lots of water. By the third trimester any skin problems should clear up. But, as always, don't worry if they don't. Remember that what is happening is amazing and so are you.

Breathlessness

This is very common in pregnancy. Hormonal changes cause you to breathe more deeply, which can feel like breathlessness. As your baby gets bigger it also puts pressure on your lungs, reducing their capacity, so you get out of breath more easily.

What to do: This goes away once you've given birth, but in the meantime, take it easy and don't push yourself too hard.

Snoring

Higher levels of the hormone estrogen can cause a swelling in the nose lining which can lead to snoring. Increased blood flow also causes a swelling in the nose and excessive weight gain can make the problem worse.

What to do: Try to stick to the recommended weight gain during your pregnancy and sleep on your left side.

ON THE PLUS SIDE...

It's not all bad news: as well as experiencing some unpleasant pregnancy symptoms, you may also be discovering some definite perks!

SHINY, THICK HAIR

During pregnancy your hair may look thicker, bouncier, and more shiny. It's not that you're growing any more hair—just that you're not losing any; you may well have noticed that it's not falling out during hair washes or brushing. An increased blood flow to the scalp can also result in shinier locks.

GLOWING SKIN

Increased blood flow brings more blood to the face, giving you a smoother complexion. Plus, if you cut out alcohol (which should be a pregnancy given) and sugary foods, your skin will glow even more.

FULLER BREASTS

Even before your milk comes in your breasts may look fuller and firmer and you can go up a cup size or two.

STRONG NAILS

Hormone changes will make your nails grow faster and stronger.

STAYING SAFE THROUGHOUT YOUR PREGNANCY

You'll be bombarded with advice in your pregnancy, some true, some not so true. Here's everything you need to know. And if you're unsure about anything, speak to your midwife or doctor.

Hot tubs, saunas, and steam rooms: Some studies suggest that water at over 100°F can be damaging to developing cells. This is especially true in the first trimester. Becoming too hot can also slow down blood flow to the baby because blood flows to the surface of the skin instead to cool you down. You're also more likely to become dehydrated. So avoid hot tubs, saunas, and steam rooms throughout your whole pregnancy and make sure your baths at home aren't too hot either.

Cats: There is often some confusion about cats and pregnancy. In a nutshell, it's perfectly safe to be around cats as long as you follow a few guidelines. Toxoplasmosis is caused by a parasite called *Toxoplasma gondii* that can be found in cat feces (as well as in undercooked meat and sheep). If you develop toxoplasmosis in pregnancy, it can be harmful to your baby and increase your risk of miscarriage and stillbirth. However, it's important to note that this is very rare. Avoid emptying cat-litter boxes or wear rubber gloves if you do. Also wear gloves while gardening (to avoid cat feces), avoid sheep, and wash your hands thoroughly if you touch a cat or a sheep.

Cleaning products: Relatively little is known about the effects of cleaning products on pregnant women; however, I'd advise you to err on the side of caution because your baby absorbs what you absorb. Avoid big jobs like cleaning the oven, as oven cleaners let off a lot of fumes. If you do use products like cleaning sprays and air fresheners, keep the windows open so air circulates. Better still, opt for a natural cleaning product that doesn't use chemicals. For example, a company I love called e-cloth makes cloths in which microfibers trap dirt and grime using just water, without any need for chemical cleaners. They're great for you and the environment, because you're not flushing cleaning chemicals down the bath or sink.

Paint fumes: Before the 1970s, lead elements were found in paint which were shown to be harmful to unborn babies. Although the risks from popular household paints today are very low, why take the chance? Don't schedule decorating during your pregnancy and, if you do, stay away from the paint and keep doors and windows open. Also avoid eating, drinking, or sleeping in a room that's recently been painted.

Pollution: A 2013 study from the Harvard School of Public Health found that pregnant women exposed to high levels of pollution were up to twice as likely to have a child with autism. However, it's important to remember that they were exposed to high levels. Walking along a busy road won't do you any harm and millions of women who live in big, smoky cities have healthy babies. However, it's worth trying to avoid pollution where possible—so if you walk to work along a busy road, switch to a greener route if you can.

Smoking: If you're currently pregnant, I'm sure you don't smoke; the fact that you're reading this book means that you care about your health and that of your baby, but I want to cover everything here, so this is a quick reminder that it's absolutely not OK—ever—to smoke during pregnancy. Anything that you eat, drink or inhale gets into your baby's bloodstream, including cigarette smoke, which contains thousands of chemicals, many of which can cause cancer. Nicotine and carbon monoxide are two of the most harmful chemicals and can cause miscarriage, premature birth, and low birthweight. Nicotine also reduces your baby's oxygen supply and studies have found that babies whose mothers smoked during pregnancy are more likely to have a heart defect and lungs that do not develop properly, and there is also more chance that they will have a low IQ, behavioral problems, and developmental delays. Plus, smoking can reduce your fertility by 40 percent, so if you are trying to conceive, quit as soon as possible.

If you're struggling to give up smoking, speak to your doctor or midwife immediately and ask them for information on how to quit, including courses and self-help techniques. Now is the time to focus on your own and your baby's health. You both deserve a happy, healthy life.

C&L FOODS FOR PREGNANCY

IT'S WORTH REMEMBERING:

✻ You need to cook fish, meat, and poultry thoroughly, so they're piping hot throughout with no trace of pink or blood.
✻ Cook your eggs well, so the white and yolk are solid. For this reason it's better to have scrambled eggs or omelets rather than poached eggs, which can be runny.
✻ Be extra vigilant about washing fruits and vegetables.
✻ Have only pasteurized milk, yogurt, and cheese.
✻ Continue taking a 400 mcg supplement of folic acid for the first 12 weeks of pregnancy, and a 15 mcg supplement of vitamin D throughout pregnancy and breastfeeding.
✻ Limit yourself to two portions of oily fish a week. They can contain high levels of mercury, which can be harmful to your baby's developing nervous system.

AND AVOID THE FOLLOWING:

✻ Pâtés – whether fish, meat, or vegetable, they are more likely than other foods to contain listeria bacteria, which cause listeriosis (a type of food poisoning) and you're more susceptible to it when you're pregnant because your immune system is weaker. Listeriosis is usually a mild illness, but it can harm your baby and cause premature birth and even miscarriage—it's very rare, but why take the risk?
✻ Mold-ripened soft cheese, such as brie and camembert, and blue-veined cheeses such as Danish blue and gorgonzola—they're also more likely to contain listeria.
✻ Foods containing raw or undercooked eggs, like fresh mayonnaise; store-bought is fine as it's pasteurized.
✻ Marlin, swordfish, or shark, as they contain high levels of mercury.
✻ Raw shellfish, such as oysters or mussels, because they can contain bacteria that may cause food poisoning.
✻ Liver and liver products – they contain a lot of vitamin A, which can harm a developing baby. For the same reason, don't take fish liver oil or other supplements that contain vitamin A.

FOODS YOU CAN EAT DURING PREGNANCY:

✻ Sushi – it's fine to eat sushi made with raw fish, as long as the fish used to make it has been frozen first. Raw fish can contain parasitic worms that could cause food poisoning, but freezing kills them. So buy sushi from well-established restaurant chains and ask them if their fish has been frozen. You can also opt for vegetarian sushi.
✻ Peanuts – peanuts and peanut butter are fine, as long as you don't have a nut allergy.
✻ Hard cheeses, like Cheddar and Parmesan.
✻ Soft cheeses – as long as they're made from pasteurized milk (check the label), it's safe to eat cream cheese, goat cheese, mozzarella, and halloumi.

ALWAYS KEEP THESE IN YOUR HOME:

Fresh fruit - you can grab a piece whenever you feel hungry, rather than heading for the cookie jar.
A lemon - squeeze it over salads to add flavor or add a slice to cold water for a refreshing drink, or to warm water (boiled and then cooled) to flush out your system.
A bag of unsalted nuts - grab a handful to keep you going when you haven't had time to cook.
Avocados - the perfect snack, full of healthy, filling fats; and the creamy texture will satisfy a sweet tooth. Slice half of one over some gluten-free crackers.
Eggs - two scrambled eggs on rye bread or an omelet filled with whatever vegetables you have in your fridge make a nutritious, filling meal, whether it's breakfast or dinner.
Something green - always try to have something green with your meals, such as avocado, green bell pepper, green apples, spinach, arugula, or broccoli.

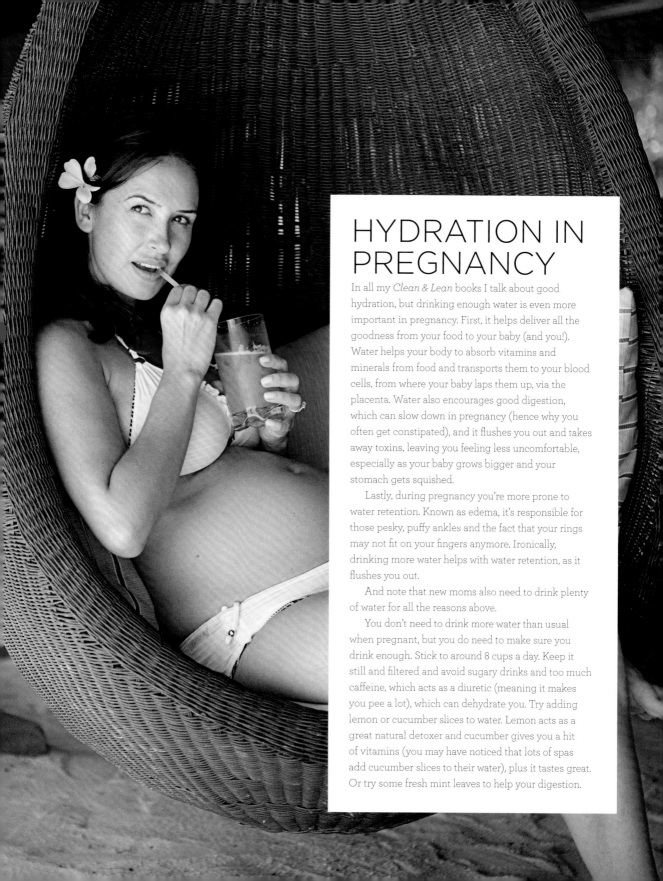

HYDRATION IN PREGNANCY

In all my *Clean & Lean* books I talk about good hydration, but drinking enough water is even more important in pregnancy. First, it helps deliver all the goodness from your food to your baby (and you!). Water helps your body to absorb vitamins and minerals from food and transports them to your blood cells, from where your baby laps them up, via the placenta. Water also encourages good digestion, which can slow down in pregnancy (hence why you often get constipated), and it flushes you out and takes away toxins, leaving you feeling less uncomfortable, especially as your baby grows bigger and your stomach gets squished.

Lastly, during pregnancy you're more prone to water retention. Known as edema, it's responsible for those pesky, puffy ankles and the fact that your rings may not fit on your fingers anymore. Ironically, drinking more water helps with water retention, as it flushes you out.

And note that new moms also need to drink plenty of water for all the reasons above.

You don't need to drink more water than usual when pregnant, but you do need to make sure you drink enough. Stick to around 8 cups a day. Keep it still and filtered and avoid sugary drinks and too much caffeine, which acts as a diuretic (meaning it makes you pee a lot), which can dehydrate you. Try adding lemon or cucumber slices to water. Lemon acts as a great natural detoxer and cucumber gives you a hit of vitamins (you may have noticed that lots of spas add cucumber slices to their water), plus it tastes great. Or try some fresh mint leaves to help your digestion.

EXERCISE DURING PREGNANCY

If your pregnancy is normal and you feel fine and up to it, moderate exercise at this stage can help you feel better, but don't feel pressured. Just being active and walking every day is also fine.

There are several benefits of exercise during pregnancy. It can:
✳ ease or prevent back pain and other discomforts (as long as you do it correctly—and in this book I'll show you how)
✳ boost your mood and energy levels
✳ help you sleep better
✳ help prevent excess weight gain—you shouldn't be worrying about your weight in pregnancy, but nor do you need to be gaining an excessive amount
✳ increase stamina and muscle strength
✳ help prevent orthopedic issues, such as back and knee pain
✳ reduce the risk of pre- and postnatal depression
✳ make giving birth easier
✳ improve your ability to deal with labor—the fitter you are, the better you'll be able to cope (trust me, this will come in handy)
✳ help reduce constipation, which is a common pregnancy side effect, plus it reduces swelling and bloating
✳ possibly prevent or help gestational diabetes.

However, as with everything else pregnancy-related, listen to your body at all times and check with your health practitioner or midwife before exercising. If you feel unwell, breathless, or as if you can't carry on at any point, stop immediately. Don't push yourself.

It's best to continue exercising in a similar manner to the way you did before you got pregnant. For example, if you ran regularly and went to the gym every week, continue with this, but listen to your body and slow things down if you need to.

If you rarely exercised before you got pregnant, don't take it up now in the hope of keeping your weight down. Instead, start slowly with walking and swimming and find a local yoga or Pilates class that specializes in pregnancy.

Stop any risky or high-impact sports, such as horse riding, hockey, tennis, scuba diving, ice skating, or hiking at high altitudes. Check with your midwife or OB about skiing and road biking.

Stop exercising immediately if you experience any of the following (and if the symptoms don't pass, call the maternity unit at your hospital or your doctor):
✳ feeling faint or dizziness
✳ increased shortness of breath
✳ chest pain
✳ headache
✳ muscle weakness
✳ calf pain or swelling

If any of the following happens, call the maternity unit at your hospital or your doctor immediately:
✳ contractions, even if they're mild and irregular
✳ vaginal bleeding
✳ decreased fetal movement in the later stages of pregnancy (you usually feel your baby's first movements at around weeks 17 or 18, although sometimes earlier with second or third pregnancies)
✳ fluid leaking from the vagina

TOP TIPS FOR EXERCISE DURING PREGNANCY

✳ Avoid brisk exercise in hot, humid weather.

✳ Wear comfortable clothing that will help you stay cool.

✳ Wear a non-underwire bra that fits well and gives lots of support. It's a good idea to have your bra size professionally measured two or three times during pregnancy to ensure that you're wearing a bra that protects your growing breasts.

✳ Drink plenty of water to keep you hydrated (see p. 61).

✳ Monitor your heart rate; aim to keep it no higher than 140bpm.

✳ Stop any time you feel as though you can't go on. Remember, listen to your body.

EXERCISE IN THE FIRST TRIMESTER:

Perform the workout below 3–4 times a week on non-consecutive days. On the days between your workouts, go for a brisk walk or a light swim. Your workouts should last no longer than 30–45 minutes and, as always, ensure that you listen to your body and take plenty of rest between sets.

Perform each exercise, one after the other, until you have performed all the exercises in the circuit, then rest for 60 seconds. Between each exercise, take 30–60 seconds rest, depending on how you are feeling. Perform the whole circuit of exercises 2–3 times.

EXERCISE	REPS	SETS	REST
Tummy vacuum	8–10	2–3	30–60 secs
Hip extension	15	2–3	30–60 secs
Side-lying single-leg knee-raise with mini-band	8–10/side	2–3	30–60 secs
Mini-band walking	10 steps/side	2–3	30–60 secs
Y	10–15	2–3	30–60 secs
Squat	12–15	2–3	30–60 secs
T	15	2–3	30–60 secs
Superman	12–15/side	2–3	60 secs
Hip abduction	12–15/side	2–3	60 secs

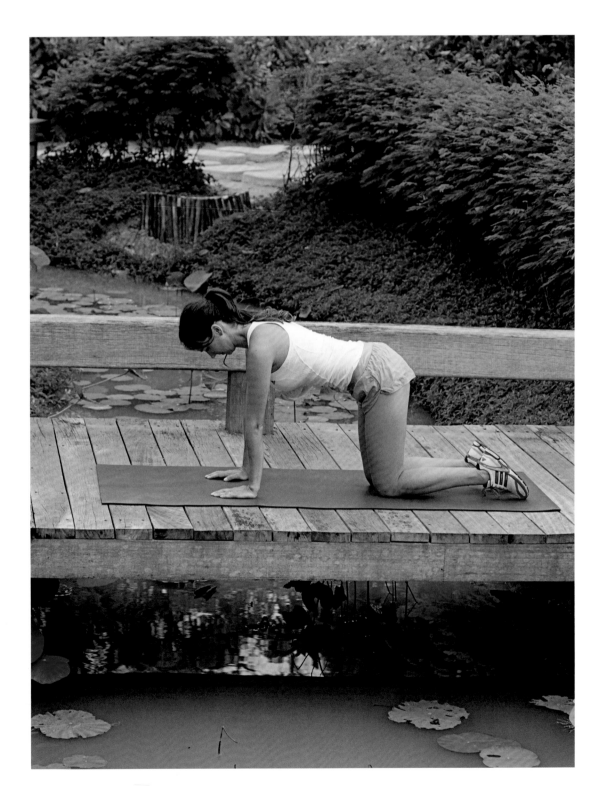

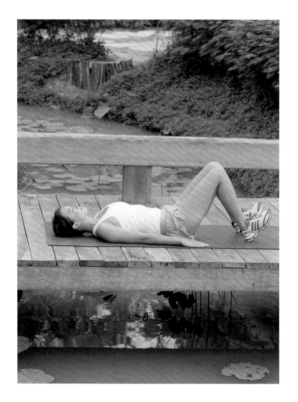

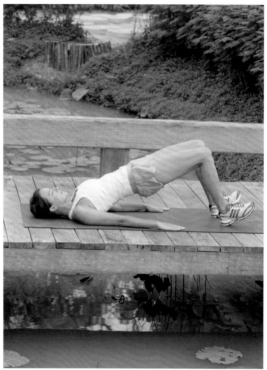

Hip extension

Start position: Lie on your back with both knees bent and heels on the ground. Point your toes up to the ceiling and place your arms by your sides.

The movement: Lift your hips off the ground, raising them as high as you can go, squeezing the glutes (your butt muscles, which help protect your lower back). Pause at the top for 1 second, then return to the start position. Repeat 15 times.

Opposite:

Tummy vacuum

Start position: Support yourself on your hands and knees with hands under shoulders, arms straight, and knees under hips. Make sure your arms and thighs remain at right angles to the floor, keep your back straight, and keep your head aligned with your upper back.

The movement: Relax your stomach, letting it sag toward the floor while maintaining a flat back. Then squeeze your tummy muscles and pull your belly button toward the ceiling, still maintaining a flat back. Repeat 8–10 times.

*top tip

This is great for your bottom and lower back. Place a Bodyism mini-band (bodyism.com) around your legs, just above your knees, for added resistance!

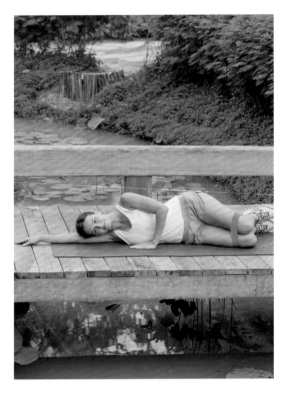
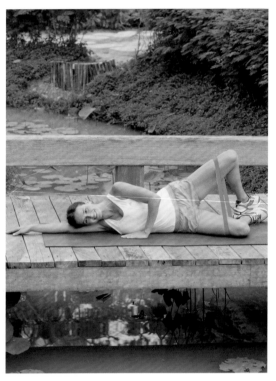

Side-lying single-leg knee-raise with mini-band

Start position: Place a Bodyism mini-band around both legs just above your knees. Lie on your right side with your right arm extended, palm facing down, and rest your head on your arm. Bend your knees to a 90-degree angle and stack them on top of one another. Keep your body in line and engage your core by pulling your belly button in toward your spine.

The movement: Raise your top knee by pushing against the resistance of the mini-band. Take the knee up as far as you can without straining the lower back, keeping both feet together. With control, slowly lower back to the start position. Repeat 8–10 times on each side.

*top tip

Make sure your head is supported to create the most comfortable position for your body to be in, as well as maintaining good posture.

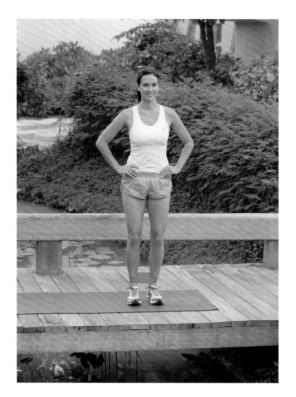
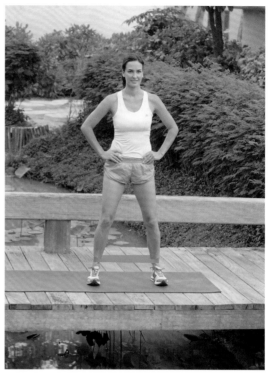

Mini-band walking

Start position: Take a Bodyism mini-band of your chosen strength and place it just above your ankles. Stand with your feet hip-width apart, hands resting on your hips and engage the core by pulling your belly button in toward your spine.

The movement: Take one large step out sideways to the right, keeping the legs straight and without using your body for momentum. Then bring your left foot in half a step, keeping tension in the band all the time. Repeat this movement for 10 steps on each side.

*top tip

This exercise strengthens and lifts your bottom like nothing else. It will also ensure your lower back stays strong and healthy throughout your pregnancy.

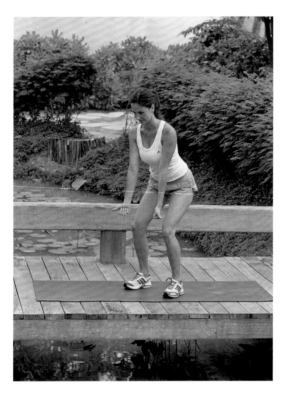
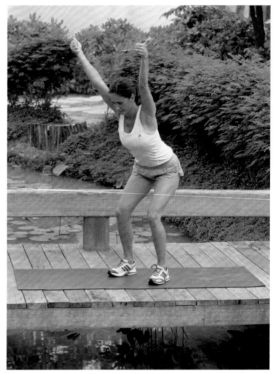

Y

Start position: Stand with your feet hip-width apart, bend
your knees, and stick your bottom out, so your upper body
leans forward 45 degrees. Hold your hands directly below
your chest with fists clenched and thumbs up, keeping
your head and back all in a straight line, your shoulders
back and down. Engage your core by pulling your belly
button in toward the spine.

The movement: Raise both hands to create a "Y" shape
above your head with your arms by your ears, then return
to the starting point. Repeat 10–15 times.

*top tip
This exercise will strengthen
your shoulders and upper back.
Perform the movement slowly to
make sure your posture remains
good throughout your pregnancy.

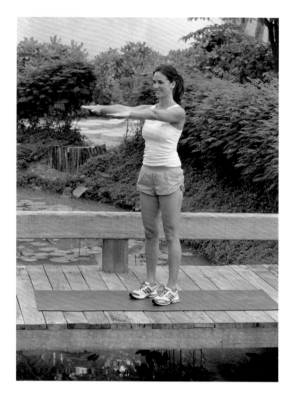

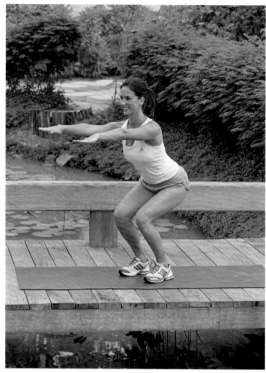

Squat

Start position: Take a comfortable stance with your feet shoulder-width apart, toes pointing forward and arms out in front of you, level with your chest. Engage your core by pulling your belly button in toward the spine.

The movement: Initiate the squat by bending the knees and by pushing the hips back. Squat back and down until the thighs are parallel to the floor. Keep your arms straight. Return to the standing position by pushing through the heels. Do not let the knees collapse inward during the movement, keep the arms extended in front of your chest, and keep your chest up and your back flat. Repeat 12–15 times.

*top tip

This is a great lower-body toner that improves balance and energy flow. It helps relax the pelvic-floor muscles, creating more room in the pelvis which can, in turn, make pregnancy, labor, and childbirth more comfortable.

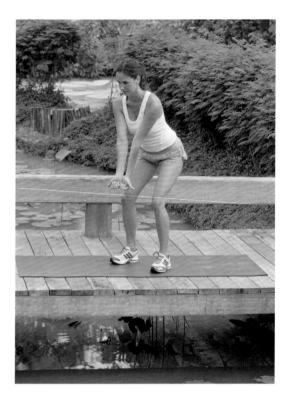 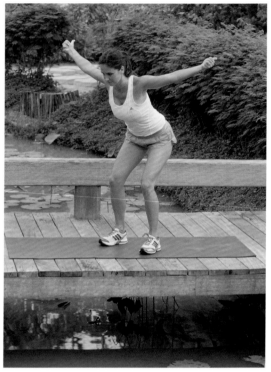

T

Start position: Stand with your feet hip-width apart.
Bend your knees and lean forward so your torso is at a
45-degree angle. Keep your head and back all in a straight
line, your shoulders back and down, and your hands
directly below your chest with fists clenched and thumbs
pointing outward. Engage your core by pulling your belly
button in toward the spine.

The movement: Keeping your body still and your core
engaged, raise your arms out to the sides to form a "T"
shape, then return to the start position. Repeat 15 times.

*top tip
This exercise will strengthen your
upper back—perfect if you have
found your posture deteriorating
during your pregnancy.

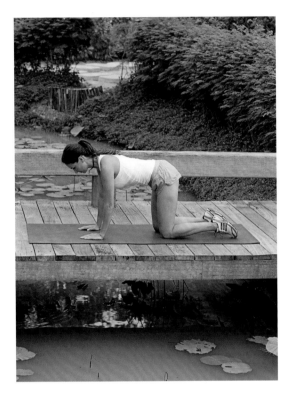 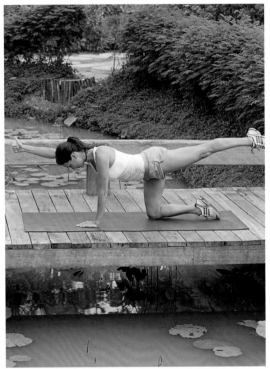

Superman

Start position: Support yourself on your hands and knees with hands under shoulders and knees under hips and with your toes firmly pointed into the floor. Make sure your spine and neck are in a straight line by keeping your gaze to the floor, just in front of your fingertips.

The movement: Extend your right arm out in front of you beyond your head, thumb up, while extending your left leg backward—imagine you are being pulled from either end. Return to the start position and repeat 12–15 times on each side.

*top tip

This exercise will activate and strengthen your hamstrings, glutes, and lower-back muscles, as well as improving your overall body balance. It is also one of the safest movements to help strengthen your back throughout your pregnancy.

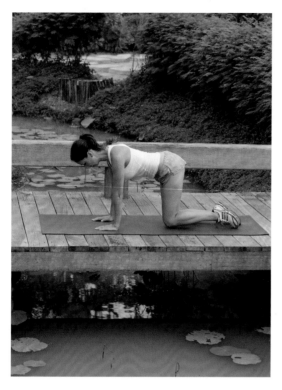 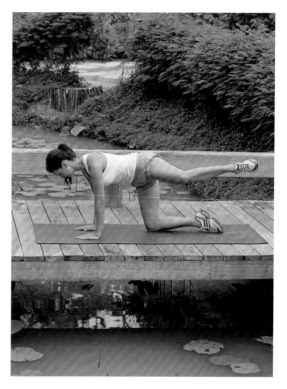

Hip abduction

Start position: Support yourself on all fours with hands under shoulders and knees under hips. Make sure your arms and thighs remain at right angles to the floor, keeping your back straight and your head aligned with your upper back. Draw your bellybutton in toward your spine to engage the core.

The movement: Keeping your upper body still—a flat back and straight arms—slowly lift your left knee to the side and slightly back, while keeping the knee bent throughout the movement. Then slowly return to the start position and repeat 12–15 times before moving on to the opposite leg.

*top tip

This exercise is great for strengthening and toning the glutes (your butt muscles, which help protect your lower back). Perform the movement slowly and keep your breathing regular to keep your body calm and not stressed.

YOGA FOR PREGNANCY

Wenche Beard is an amazing lady and yoga expert whom we've worked with for years. She designed a wonderful program that nurtured Christiane throughout her pregnancy and I'm so happy she is able to share her wisdom here. Wenche says:

"Pregnancy is a magical experience and you should celebrate the life growing inside you. When you're pregnant and practicing yoga, it gives you the opportunity to connect with your changing body and your growing baby. In the busy-ness of life, moms-to-be need some time to stop and connect with themselves in a deeper way.

"During pregnancy your body goes through some tremendous changes as it evolves to accommodate your growing baby. In my experience of working with pregnant women, I've found that they should practice yoga asanas [postures] to stay strong and in the best possible shape.

"Yoga won't just give you a healthy body, but a healthy mind too, helping you to balance your emotions through the hormonal and physical changes that are taking place. Yoga asanas and pranayama [breath control] can help prevent common pregnancy ailments such as sickness, shortness of breath, heartburn, swollen ankles, and sciatica. It also helps you prepare for the birth as it enables you to 'tune in' to your body and assists with better breathing techniques. Before practicing yoga during pregnancy, always consult your prenatal health-care provider, doctor, or midwife for advice.

"When you practice yoga in pregnancy you practice yoga with your baby at the very center of your body and your baby will always from now on be at the very center of your life. *Namaste.*"

BY WENCHE BEARD, *British Wheel of Yoga teacher*

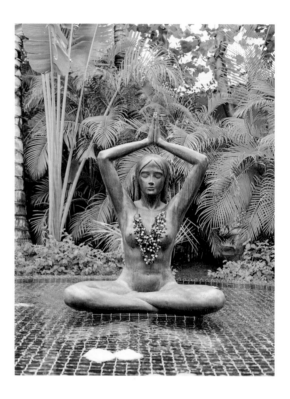

*top tip

If you are going to do yoga during pregnancy, please be careful to make sure your instructor is qualified for pregnancy yoga. Get references and follow your instincts.

Yoga moves for your first trimester

"Major changes are taking place during these first three months of your pregnancy. This is the trimester where your fetus is implanting itself into your uterus. And even though it's tiny, already at ten weeks your little one is wriggling and moving about even though you won't be able to feel it for several more weeks yet.

"I'm often asked, 'Should I practice yoga in the first trimester?' If you're a healthy and active woman, and you've been practicing yoga for a while, the answer is yes, although you may want to adjust your routine slightly. If you're new to yoga, it's often recommended to wait until you're twelve weeks pregnant before starting. I always recommend that clients speak to their health-care provider or doctor as soon as they discover they're pregnant for advice on exercise. In most cases your doctor will be happy for you to get onto the yoga mat."

HERE ARE WENCHE'S YOGA-IN-PREGNANCY PRECAUTIONS:

✱ Avoid stretching your muscles too much, especially your stomach muscles.
✱ Be careful in standing poses as gravity and balance change. Use supports such as blocks, walls, or sturdy tables.
✱ Avoid deep belly twists.
✱ Avoid deep back bends.
✱ Avoid sharp movements.
✱ Avoid holding asanas (postures) for too long.
✱ Listen to your body at all times and stop if you feel uncomfortable.

Breathing/pranayama

"Pranayama, the 'yogic breath,' is a deeper, more controlled breath. 'Prana' means energy and 'ayama' means distributing energy. When we breathe in, we inhale oxygen and prana (life energy); this is vital for the functioning of your body and the healthy growth of your baby. As we breathe out, we release carbon dioxide and other impurities the body doesn't need. The breath is a vital part of life, and when you are breathing well, your baby is breathing well too."

The breath control

"Get comfortable in a seated position, keeping your arms relaxed and your hands resting in your lap. Or in the 'gyan mudra' (where your arms are straight, with the back of your hands on your knees and your index finger and thumb touching—this is the most common hand position in meditation and some pranayama practices). Or keep your hands on your abdomen, cradling your baby and feeling the rise and fall of your belly as you breathe. The breathing technique is known as Ujjayi breathing, and is often referred to as the 'ocean breath,' because the sound at the back of the throat resembles that of the ocean. When you practice this breath, there is a slight contraction of the vocal cords as you breathe in and out through the nose deeply, keeping your jaw, face, shoulders, and belly relaxed. Breathe in fully and exhale completely, drinking the life force available to you and your baby, oxygenating your blood flow, making your blood purer, strengthening your lungs, enhancing your energy levels, balancing your nervous system, and creating a sense of better wellbeing.

"The simple technique of Ujjayi breathing can also help during the physical and emotional demands of labor and birth. When you're fearful or in pain, your body produces the stress hormone adrenaline and produces less of the feel-good hormone oxytocin, which facilitates birth and makes labor progress. The more relaxed your body is, the easier the birth."

Opposite are some moves to begin with.

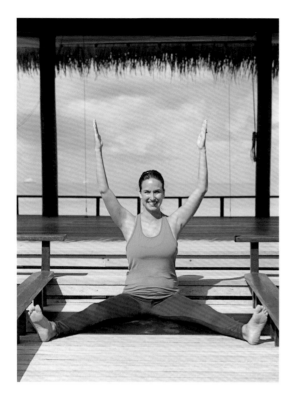

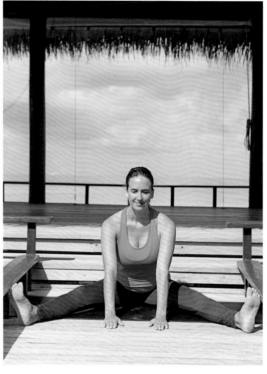

Upavistha Konasana (Wide-angle seated forward bend)

Sit on the floor with your legs as wide apart as you can comfortably get them. Tilt your pelvis, so that you sit on your "sitting bones."

Let the spine rise from the floor, and move the top of your head toward the sky. Lift your arms above your head, so your fingers face the sky as you inhale.

As you exhale, extend the body forward into the forward bend, lengthening the torso. Bring your hands on to the floor and relax your shoulders. Stay for 6–9 healthy breaths.

*top tip

This is a gentle stretch for the hips and lower back, which can become tight during pregnancy. Remember that it's important you don't strain yourself, so stretch only as far as is comfortable and keep movements relaxed and fluid.

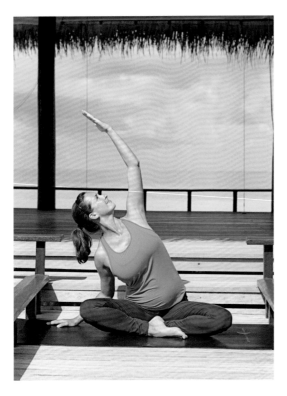 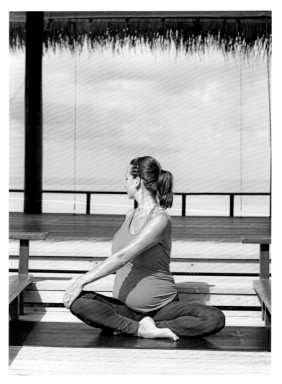

Sukhasana side stretch (Easy pose side stretch)

Sit cross-legged on the floor (or with your legs wide, if you prefer) with your arms by your sides.

Practice a long spine and place your right hand on the floor. As you inhale, let the left hand rise to the sky along the left side of the body.

As you exhale, slowly lean over to the right side and lift and rotate your upper chest, gazing upward at the sky. Stay for 3–6 breaths, breathing into the left side of your body. Come back to the center on an inhale and repeat on the other side.

Sukhasana twist (Cross-legged seated upper-spinal twist)

Sit cross-legged on the floor (or with your legs wide, if you prefer), with your spine tall; place your left hand on your right knee and rest the right hand on the floor behind you.

Inhale through the length of your spine, then exhale and let the exhalation take you into this gentle upper spinal twist. Stay for 3–6 breaths, keeping the crown of your head high to the sky and your chest wide.

Come back to the center on an inhale. Exhale, digesting the benefits before repeating on the other side.

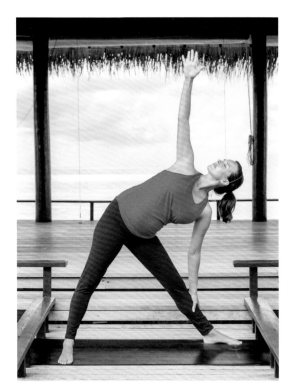

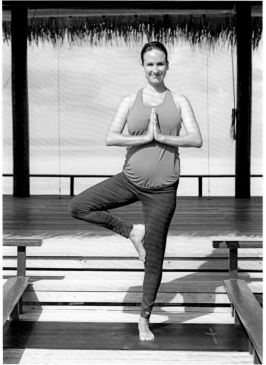

Trikonasana (Triangle pose)

Stand tall, aware of your baby at the very center of your body, then walk your feet about 3 feet or so apart. Place your hands on your hips and turn your right foot 90 degrees, aligning your right heel with your left instep, hips level to the front.

Drop your arms by the side of your body and, as you inhale, lift the arms out to the side, parallel to the floor. Then, as you exhale, draw back through the left hip as you extend your torso over your left leg with an open waist. (Support yourself on your leg, blocks, or even a chair if you need to.) Reach up to the sky with your right arm, keeping your neck long and remembering your head is an extension of the spine.

Lengthen the tailbone toward your right heel, keep the legs strong, the spine long, and arms active. Stay for 3–6 breaths, then come back on an inhale and lower the arms on the exhale. Take a few breaths here with your hands on your belly, embodying the state of balance for both you and your baby. Repeat on the other side.

Vrksasana (Tree pose)

Stand tall, imagining roots growing into the earth from the base of your feet, like a tree. Transfer weight into the left foot and lift the right leg, placing the foot, toes pointing down, on the inside of your left thigh. Bring your hands into prayer position at your heart center, pressing your palms together and lifting your sternum to the thumbs, creating space for your baby and your internal organs.

Keep your gaze focused on one point and when you are stable, raise the arms up so your hands are parallel, palms facing. Lengthen the crown of the head, relax your shoulders, and keep your standing leg strong. Here you become the tree of life—feel yourself strong and balanced, reaching to your highest potential and breathe well for 3–6 breaths.

When you are ready to come out, inhale and, as you exhale, place your palms together in prayer position above your head, then draw your hands down through your center, and come back to your heart. Release your leg and take a few moments standing tall with one hand on your heart and one on your belly feeling truly blessed. Repeat on the other side.

MISCARRIAGE

A miscarriage is the loss of a baby before twenty-four weeks. It can be an extremely distressing experience and, sadly, early miscarriages (before twelve weeks) are very common. Some studies suggest that one in four pregnancies results in miscarriage. Often women don't even know they've miscarried, especially if they weren't trying for a baby or if they have an irregular cycle. Late miscarriages (after twelve weeks) are much rarer.

Nobody really knows what causes a miscarriage, but experts think that it's usually due to the baby not developing as it should or health issues with the mother, such as a problem with the placenta. The only lifestyle factors that will increase your risk are things like smoking, alcohol, excessive amounts of caffeine, and illegal drugs.

Nearly all of you will know somebody who has had a miscarriage. While we were writing this book my wife Christiane suffered one. Here's her story.

CHRISTIANE'S STORY

"Charlotte was nine months old when we felt ready to try for another baby. I felt like my body was strong enough, I'd recovered from pregnancy and childbirth, and I was finally getting some sleep. In July 2012 I missed a period and took a test right away that came back positive. Because we'd struggled for so long to conceive Charlotte, we were very excited and told our friends and family right away. Knowing that Charlotte was soon going to have a little brother or sister to play with made me so happy. Because my pregnancy with her had been straightforward and because I'm a positive person, I just expected everything to be OK.

"I had a scan at around eight weeks and at first the doctor said the baby didn't look big enough. Then they told us the devastating news that they couldn't find a heartbeat. They thought it had happened at around seven weeks. A week later I had the most awful cramping and bleeding as I miscarried our baby. I was crushed, and looked for a reason. Was it that yoga class I took or all the traveling we'd been doing? I think women often look for a reason for these things and blame themselves, but my doctor reassured me it was 'just one of those things.' It's often just the body's way of not going through with an unhealthy pregnancy or baby.

"Luckily I had James's support, and having to get up each day and care for Charlotte helped enormously—looking after her helped take my mind off things and kept me busy. That's not to say I wasn't devastated. I so badly wanted another baby, not just for us, but for Charlotte too. And a close friend announced her pregnancy soon after and her due date was the same as mine would have been. That was incredibly tough. But I've tried to stay positive and I've told myself things happen in life for a reason. Sometimes that reason is hard to see, but it all becomes apparent in time. I trust in the universe and my body. And I know that little soul will come back to us again some day in another baby and I can't wait."